Praise for *The Toxin Solution*

"Dr. Pizzorno's *The Toxin Solution* is
exploding burden of environmental to
ing autoimmunity, obesity, cancer, and
toxins and disease is now as undisputed........ by the medical
community. For the first time, we have a clear road map of how these
toxins impact our health, but more importantly, a practical plan for
reducing our exposures and maximizing our body's own detoxification.
This book should be a mandatory part of all medical school curricu-
lums. And for any human living in the 21st century seeking to improve
their health, this book is essential reading."

> —Mark Hyman, MD, director of the Cleveland Clinic Center for
> Functional Medicine; #1 *New York Times* bestselling author of
> *Eat Fat, Get Thin*; Pritzker Foundation chair in Functional Medicine,
> Cleveland Clinic Lerner College of Medicine; founder and medical
> director of The UltraWellness Center; and chairman of the Institute for
> Functional Medicine

"We have been waiting for this groundbreaking book, *The Toxin Solution*,
from natural medicine leader Dr. Joseph Pizzorno. There has been the
need for a person of his stature and understanding of the field to separate the fact from the fiction as it relates to toxicity and detoxification.
This important book provides information that only an expert in the
field could compile and describe in a such an understandable way that it
takes the discussion of toxicity from theoretical to actionable. This is a
must read for anyone seriously interested in how environmental toxins
influence human health and what a person can do to reduce their body
burden of these disease-producing chemicals."

> —Jeffrey Bland, PhD, FACN, president of the Personalized Lifestyle
> Medicine Institute, founder of *Functional Medicine,* and author of
> *The Disease Delusion*

"Surprising and disturbing, and also illuminating and hopeful. Dr.
Pizzorno, a world-renowned authority on natural medicine, presents

cutting-edge research that shows how the toxins in our environment and our food make us ill. He gives us clear, easy-to-follow guidelines for reversing the process and restoring and enhancing our health."

—James S. Gordon, MD, former chair of the White House Commission on Complementary and Alternative Medicine Policy and author of *Unstuck: Your Guide to the Seven-Stage Journey Out of Depression*

"*The Toxin Solution* is another seminal contribution from the mind of an enormously insightful healer and thought leader. While extremely provocative, it is also quite practical in providing answers to some of our biggest health challenges. It may also provide the tipping point leading to needed changes in food production, agriculture, and environmental policies."

—Michael T. Murray, ND

"It's a given that each and every one of us is threatened by a challenging array of environmental toxins, day in and day out. In *The Toxin Solution,* Dr. Joseph Pizzorno's decades of experience are utilized to create a powerful guide to dramatically reduce our exposure to worrisome substances that are now recognized as playing central roles in chronic diseases. Even more importantly, he empowers the reader with strategies designed to enhance our ability to offload the burden of toxins that we've accumulated, allowing health to flourish."

—David Perlmutter, MD, author of the #1 *New York Times* bestseller *Grain Brain* and *The Grain Brain Whole Life Plan*

"Dr. Joseph Pizzorno has crafted a welcome examination of the man-made world and its effects on our health and longevity. Clearly and engagingly written, this book does not shy away from data and scientific evidence, which is presented in a balanced and straightforward manner. Of particular value is a gift that only a seasoned clinician can provide: An abundance of helpful and effective prescriptive advice. A much-needed and timely addition to your self-help library."

—Peter D'Adamo, ND, distinguished professor of Clinical Sciences, University of Bridgeport, and author of *Eat Right 4 Your Type*

THE
TOXIN
Solution

**How Hidden Poisons in the Air, Water, Food,
and Products We Use Are Destroying Our Health—
AND WHAT WE CAN DO TO FIX IT**

JOSEPH PIZZORNO, ND

HarperOne
An Imprint of HarperCollins*Publishers*

I dedicate *The Toxin Solution* to the courageous pioneers who kept this medicine alive despite over a century of oppression by the vested interests of conventional medicine. The foundational naturopathic medicine concepts of nutrition and detoxification are now even more important in our modern world of nutrient-depleted foods and overwhelming environmental pollution. I continue to find quite remarkable how research has finally proven the validity and efficacy of these concepts, which were once mocked, and whose practitioners were imprisoned. They are now understood to be the only solution to the health-care crisis.

And finally, I dedicate this book to you, the readers, who are no longer willing to accept that the heavy burden of ill health and disease so many suffer is "normal" and are taking their health into their own hands.

HarperOne

HarperCollins books may be purchased for educational, business, or sales promotional use. For information, please email the Special Markets Department at SPsales@harpercollins.com.

FIRST HARPERCOLLINS PAPERBACK EDITION PUBLISHED IN 2018

Designed by Ad Librum

Library of Congress Cataloging-in-Publication Data is available upon request.

ISBN 978-0-06-242746-5

24 25 26 27 28 LBC 13 12 11 10 9

Contents

How to Use This Book   vii

1 How Toxins Ruin Your Health   1

2 The Causes of Toxic Overload   39

3 The Two-Week Jumpstart Diet   69

4 Clean Up Your Gut   107

5 Restore Your Liver   137

6 Revive Your Kidneys   173

7 Intense Full-Body Detox   191

8 Stay Healthy and Detoxed   201

Appendices Introduction   221

Appendix A: Conventional Lab
Tests Indicating Toxic Load   225

Appendix B: Lab Tests for
Specific Toxins   229

Appendix C: Diseases That
Indicate Specific Toxins   231

Appendix D: Symptoms That
Indicate Specific Toxins   235

Appendix E: Symptom Tracking   239

Appendix F: Safe Products   243

Appendix G: Other Resources   245

Appendix H: Protocol Summary   247

Acknowledgments   251

References   253

Index   265

How to Use This Book

The Toxin Solution will help you learn why toxins are now the primary cause of chronic disease and what you can do to get them out of your body. The book offers a four-pronged approach to accomplishing that which includes:

1. Understanding where toxins are found and how they cause disease.
2. Preparing your detoxification systems to eliminate toxins quickly and safely.
3. Undergoing intense detoxification.
4. Following simple guidelines for a toxin-free life.

Chapters 1 and 2 present in-depth scientific explanations for the necessity to avoid and eliminate toxins to support your health. However, you do not need to understand this science to follow the book's program. You can jump ahead to the programmatic chapters and follow the steps below. (Another option is to use the summary guidance in the Appendix Protocol Summary.) It's inadvisable to skip ahead to the intense detox in week 9, as you must fully prepare your body to excrete the toxins before you start releasing them from your tissues and fat stores.

Step 1. Preparation for the Nine-Week Program (Chapter 2)— The Causes of Toxic Overload

Before launching into the nine-week program, you will learn how to protect yourself and improve health by stopping new toxins from entering your body. There is little value to getting toxins out if you keep putting more in.

Step 2. Weeks 1 and 2 (Chapter 3)—The Two-Week Jumpstart Diet

During these two weeks, you focus especially on decreasing food sources of toxins, while providing the baseline nutrients you need to support a successful detox.

Step 3. Weeks 3 and 4 (Chapter 4)—Clean Up Your Gut

Due to several factors in modern life—especially the medicinal and agricultural use of antibiotics—most people have a very toxic gut that is constantly overloading the liver. During these two weeks, you will kill off the unhealthy gut bacteria, absorb the toxins they release as they die, reseed your gut with healthy bacteria, and promote gut regeneration.

Step 4. Weeks 5 and 6 (Chapter 5)—Restore Your Liver

When healthy and well-functioning, the liver eliminates the many chemicals modern life exposes us to. During these two weeks, you will take nutrients and herbs to clean out your liver and improve its detoxification function.

Step 5. Weeks 7 and 8 (Chapter 6)—Revive Your Kidneys

As the second-most-important detoxification organ, the kidneys are vulnerable to the most long-term damage from toxin exposure. Improving their function is critical for toxin elimination and long-term health. During these two weeks you will follow a very sophisticated protocol to improve blood supply to the kidneys and promote their function.

Step 6. Week 9 (Chapter 7)—Intense Full-Body Detox

Once your body is ready, you will use saunas, nutrients, and diet to release toxins from your cells and fat stores. If you become too uncomfortable, or feel sick, slow down the process. (This step can be repeated several times if needed and in the future, as long as you maintain healthy gut, liver, and kidney function.)

1

How Toxins Ruin Your Health

Despite advances in modern medicine and technology, today more than ever people are suffering from chronic illnesses through all stages of the human life cycle. In our search for health, have we missed something? Or have the challenges evolved?

For much of the twentieth century, integrative, functional, and natural medicine doctors named nutritional deficiencies and excesses as the primary causes of chronic disease. We all know about the problems of nutrient-deficient food, excessive sugar, and unhealthy fat consumption. But, starting about sixty years ago, something fundamental changed: toxins started entering our world in massive amounts. But only relatively recently has it been possible to really grasp their effects on us. This book will change that. The latest findings I'll detail in *The Toxin Solution: How Hidden Poisons in the Air, Water, Food, and Products We Use Are Destroying Our Health—AND WHAT WE CAN DO TO FIX IT* reveal that toxins are now the invisible primary drivers of countless health problems. This book will uncover those findings, while offering a time-tested program to counter these toxins and support you in lightening your toxic load to regain your health.

When I first started offering detoxification protocols, the people who came to my clinic didn't do so because they wanted to detoxify. They came because they had minor to major health problems they sought to address. No one mentioned the word *detox,* ever. Now, it seems like every other health provider offers some form of detoxification, making it very hard for people to distinguish between all of these supposed detox programs, no less figure out what is right for them. *The Toxin Solution* will provide you with a rock-solid rationale for understanding the crucial need for detox, along with a safe, scientifically validated program anyone can safely follow. In just eight weeks (nine if you follow my bonus week) my step-by-step protocol will release your own toxic load and help you rediscover your health and vitality.

Why Toxic Exposures Are Revolutionizing Health Care

Toxins damage every aspect of our physiological function and play a role in virtually all diseases. They don't act alone. They interact with other factors in our health environment and in many cases *magnify* the disruption caused by other factors. The cutting-edge research I will share with you throughout *The Toxin Solution* reveals the strong disease causations of toxic pollutants in virtually all chronic diseases—especially diabetes, heart disease, cancer, and dementia. All these diseases are increasing in every age group. This can't be simply dismissed as due to lifestyle, nutritional deficiencies, or the increasing age of the population.

I've been involved in medicine now for almost half a century—as a researcher, student, clinician, teacher, lecturer, author, and advocate at the local, state, federal, and international levels. I've taught tens of thousands of students and doctors, authored or coauthored twelve books, written over one hundred articles in peer-reviewed scientific journals, and cared for tens of thousands of patients either directly or indirectly through sophisticated corporate wellness programs that I designed and helped implement.

What I've learned over these many years is that our bodies have a tremendous capacity to remain vital, bounce back, and heal themselves. *The Toxin Solution* will offer you the proven detox and tailored protocols I've developed to restore that vitality by releasing toxic overload. You will also learn how to avoid toxins (wherever possible) as you progressively release them from your cells, tissues, fat stores, and organs.

In just eight weeks, *The Toxin Solution* will:

- Reveal how to avoid avoidable toxins.

- Strengthen and repair detox organs: the gut, liver, and kidneys.

- Support your body's normal processes for excreting toxins.

- Actively facilitate the release of toxins.

- Repair toxin-related damage.

Many people mistakenly believe that toxins are a given and there is nothing we can do about them. But that's not true. Many people don't take toxins into account when they buy food and other products. You can shield yourself and your family by making the right choices. *The Toxin Solution* will reveal specific ways you can minimize your exposure to many toxins and avoid their deleterious health effects.

Here's just one example: When you gas up your car, do you take the trouble to position yourself upwind of the fumes? If you don't bother to do that, it may be because no one has ever told you that if you can smell the fumes, that means the chemicals in the gasoline, especially benzene, are entering your body. Yes, you can greatly lessen your avoidable toxic exposure by paying attention, as in this example. Nevertheless, if you, like the majority of the population, live in a city, or are downwind from a gas station, you will constantly breathe in low levels of the benzene that is circulating in the air. Yes, it's at a lower concentration than what you inhale when gassing up your car. But it still enters your body—and does so on a nearly daily basis. The impact? Since benzene damages DNA, this chronic exposure increases the risk of cancer. You might think you are getting only a small dose during those five minutes you are pumping gas, but the problem is that the benzene you inhale joins all the other chemicals and metals you take in every day in virtually every aspect of your life.

Going through a regular day, the average person encounters a constant stream of benzene and other chemical toxins, from chemical-laden food, paint, printing ink, flame retardants, coolants, and wood-floor finishes to Scotchgard-treated clothing, cosmetics, pizza boxes and popcorn bags, and dust. These are just a few of the everyday things that contain an alphabet soup of truly harmful toxins—PCBs, PBDEs, OCPs, VOCs, EMFs, and PFCs, not to mention arsenic, cadmium, mercury, and lead.

Many of these hundreds and thousands of chemical toxins simply didn't exist prior to the mid-twentieth century. Our grandparents undoubtedly faced their own unique stressors, but they were nothing like the barrage of chemicals, heavy metals, radiation, electromagnetic frequencies, and pollution that batter people today. Although the human body has an innate capacity to detoxify itself, people now are exposed to a level of consumer, agricultural, and industrial toxins that the human organism never evolved to handle.

Acute poisoning and high levels of heavy-metal toxicity can be easier for doctors to recognize. They are most common among people with high-exposure jobs, or those who live downstream from industrial emissions (like emissions from mining, battery manufacturing, and other industries). On the other hand, chronic low-level exposures, which the majority of people experience, produce subtler and often more pervasive symptoms.

For example, the majority of Americans now carry higher bodily levels than ever before of endocrine-disrupting chemicals. A well-known one, bisphenol A (BPA), is contained in many food cans and packaging. When you eat canned soup or drink soy milk from a BPA-coated container, you increase BPA levels more than tenfold.[1] What's the health effect? The BPA acts to disrupt your endocrine system, which regulates virtually all aspects of the body's metabolism and function. The predictable result of this barrage of endocrine disruptors is a growing incidence of chronic disease and an increased rate of aging. For example, having a level of BPA in your urine above 5 µg/L (micrograms per liter) doubles your risk of diabetes, since this toxin blocks the receptor sites on the cells that insulin activates to allow sugar in.

Figure 1.1. **BPA levels by type of container**

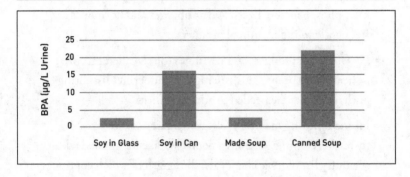

Although we now consider such nonoptimal eating patterns normal, eating canned soup every day for a week causes BPA levels over four times this threshold. Even just two servings a week doubles the risk of diabetes. Eighteen percent of the U.S. population have levels of BPA above this threshold, which also results in elevated blood pressure. And that's just one toxin.

As you will learn in this book, BPA and other toxins do all sorts of damage: they gradually clog the liver, block insulin-receptor sites, damage the genes, and undermine DNA repair and recovery. They contribute to inflammation, blood-sugar problems, digestive problems,

Figure 1.1 source: J. L. Carwile, X. Ye, X. Zhou, A. M. Calafat, and K. B. Michels, "Canned soup consumption and urinary bisphenol A: A randomized crossover trial," *Journal of the American Medical Association* 306, no. 20 (2011): 2218–20.

mitochondrial disorders, hormonal imbalances, low energy, immune issues, and a host of other problems. When toxins build up over time and overload your body, they gradually undermine your health and cause disease.

Where do toxins come from? Where are they found?

- Conventionally grown foods are sprayed with neurotoxic pesticides to kill insects; such foods are contaminated (especially GMO foods) with toxic herbicides that are sprayed to kill weeds. Rice has high arsenic levels when grown in contaminated water; heavy metals like cadmium are found in high levels in soy grown with high-phosphate fertilizers, and antibiotics and hormones are frequently found in animal products.

- Personal-care products and perfumes (often called HABAs, or health and beauty aids) are high in endocrine-disrupting phthalates that are needed to add fragrances.

- Home-building materials, cleaning materials, mattresses, furniture, clothing, and other goods we take for granted release a laundry list of toxic chemicals, the length of which continues to grow.

- Industrial activities such as gas and electrical-power production generate toxic emissions of methane, carbon dioxide, volatile organic compounds, ozone, benzene, toluene, mercury, and sulfur, contaminating the air and water around cities, suburbs, and agricultural regions. Two common chemicals emitted by gas pipelines that crisscross the country are xylene and n-hexane. Xylene can produce short-term effects like nausea and gastric discomfort. Its long-term effects include neurological problems.

As you can see from just this array of examples, exposure to the many external chemicals emitted into our world can't always be eliminated by individual avoidance. From both large-scale and small immediate sources, pollutants enter our communities, our homes, our foods, and our bodies. That is why it is so essential to understand the effects of all the toxins to which we have been exposed, learn how to avoid as many of them as possible, and increase their elimination.

Jennifer's Story

Sixty-year-old Jennifer considered herself healthy. Being proactive, she came to me for guidance on further improving her health and preventing disease. I immediately noticed that she had a pretty significant tremor. She hadn't mentioned it, she told me later, because she thought it was simply a sign of aging. Many people assume that neurodegeneration in older years is "normal." It may be common, but it's not preordained!

A basic physical exam showed a slightly underweight but otherwise healthy woman. Then I looked in her mouth and counted more than ten amalgam fillings. I immediately suspected that her tremor was due to progressive neurological damage caused by mercury leaking from her fillings. To verify that, I ran several tests. The results showed elevations of both mercury and lead.

We weren't able to identify the source of lead exposure. Most likely, lead was coming from her bones. People of Jennifer's generation and older formed a lot of their bone when lead was still being used in gasoline and paint. The bone loss triggered by menopause (and andropause) releases the metal toxins.

Since Jennifer was clearly showing damage from the lead and mercury, she decided with my encouragement to go to an ecological dentist to have the amalgams removed. She also started following my more aggressive mercury- and lead-removal support protocol—a regimen that should be undertaken only with direct medical supervision. (It's based on the all-around detox protocol you can safely do, offered later in this book.) I also encouraged her to increase her consumption of fruits and vegetables, eat only wild-caught fish, and eat more high-fiber lentils and beans.

During the first few months she suffered some symptoms, including low energy and headaches. Some people do experience symptoms when their cells start to release toxins, but Jennifer decided to stay the course. After a year, we repeated the earlier tests and found much lower levels of mercury and lead. But far more significant, her tremor was gone (so much for it being a normal sign of aging), her energy was up, and she felt much healthier and stronger.

Prior to coming to see me, Jennifer had no idea that toxic metals lodged in her body were a ticking time bomb for health problems that would one day emerge. Like her, you may be experiencing a health issue—or heading toward one—without recognizing that toxicity contributes to it. Even if you're just first experiencing very early signs of poor health, learning how to dial down your toxic overload can help resolve the issue before it goes further.

It's not just that we are all being exposed to significant levels of single toxins that are known to damage health and cause disease. The problem is that no matter where you reside in this country or world, you are immersed in a toxic soup. You are exposed to multiple toxins that work synergistically to cause even more damage and disease. A large amount of research now clearly shows that the majority of chronic disease is due to this avalanche of toxins entering our bodies intentionally and unintentionally by every possible pathway.

Yet despite this disturbing alteration of what was once a healthy and natural environment, some doctors misguidedly dismiss the need for detox. In my more than forty years of medical practice, nothing I've seen leads me to believe that the body's innate detoxification systems are capable of handling today's toxins—without the protocols described in *The Toxin Solution* that you will undertake. Many illnesses that are extremely common today are dismissed or misunderstood—like the rising incidence of neurological complaints or low-grade chronic symptoms like dementia, diabetes, fatigue, depression, and obesity. Yet many of them arise from—or are increased by—toxicity. My aim in writing *The Toxin Solution* is to guide you in providing the help your body needs in our toxic world.

The Practitioner's Journey

I am a formally trained naturopathic physician and leading educator—founding president of this country's premiere natural medicine institution, Bastyr University. I've trained generations of integrative medicine practitioners and championed natural, integrative, and functional medicine for over four decades. From my earliest years, I've had a strong orientation to evidence-based medicine. Everything I will recommend in this book, based on years of clinical experience, is scientifically validated. In fact, it has been nothing short of astounding over my lifetime to see the clinical discoveries pioneered by earlier generations of naturopathic doctors repeatedly confirmed by science. I will present many of the latest findings in this book.

But I must confess I am not yet satisfied. I would like to see even more research on the connection between toxins and disease, and on how detoxification promotes health. Nonetheless, the numbers from the new research are staggering. The research shows that toxins are far more damaging than any other known disease risk factors. Throughout this book, I will provide charts and tables to help you grasp the invisible role these toxins play in disease.

As a pioneer of integrative medicine, I'm convinced that there are three key determinants of whether or not you will enjoy health today, tomorrow, and lifelong:

1. The extent of your exposure to toxins
2. The ability of your body to neutralize or excrete toxins
3. Your commitment to building your detoxification capacity

The Toxin Solution will help you recognize the damage done by toxic exposures, while providing ways to do all of the above. My comprehensive approach entails:

- Evading avoidable toxins.
- Repairing the detox organs.

- Building detox capacity.
- Actively promoting detoxification.
- Repairing the damage.

This book is designed to support you in that fourfold plan. In chapters 1 and 2, I unveil the toxic exposures hiding in our world. By revealing the toxic burden imposed on all of us, I hope to motivate you in making a commitment to a lifestyle of detoxification, beginning with what I call the Nine-Week Program.

You will first clear the decks by avoiding the two major sources of toxins: toxin-loaded health and beauty products (which you will learn how to limit in chapter 2) and toxin-laden food. The full Nine-Week Program begins with the Two-Week Jumpstart Diet (offered in chapter 3.) This diet will convert your nutrition from toxin-laden to toxin-free, nutrient-dense foods. These two aspects of toxin avoidance (in HABAs and in food) give you a cleaner baseline for undergoing detox.

You can't detox safely or successfully if your detoxification organs are themselves toxic (or underperforming). And overburdened and dysfunctional detox organs are all too common. That's why over the next nine weeks, *The Toxin Solution* will lead you through a well-sequenced series of three two-week detox protocols that will restore each of your most essential detox organs and rebuild your detox capacity. On this scientifically validated update of the classic naturopathic approach to detox, you will progressively repair your most crucial detox organs: the gut (chapter 4), the liver (chapter 5), and the kidneys (chapter 6). During a final, ninth week of the program, you will up-level your detox using some simple but powerful techniques I will recommend.

These naturopathic methods will help you to greatly decrease your toxic load. And decreasing your toxic load makes it easier to detox. Now, instead of experiencing a downward cycle in which toxic overload progressively damages your organs and impairs your detox capacity, you will be actively creating a positive cycle by restoring your organs and rebuilding your detox capacity—by following the protocols in *The Toxin Solution*.

Naturopathic Medicine

Naturopathic medicine is built on the profound belief that the body has a tremendous ability to heal, if we just give it a chance. Naturopathic doctors specialize in helping people understand why they are sick and how to become healthy by using natural therapies. They focus on:

- Searching for the underlying causes of illness rather than suppressing symptoms.
- Following the principle of "first do no harm."
- Educating patients about self-healing, self-care, and prevention.
- Taking into account each individual's unique physical, mental, emotional, genetic, environmental, social, and other factors in an effort to treat the whole person.

Toxic Overload

While lifestyle, diet, and genetics all play a major role in your health, symptoms of declining health and chronic disease often start with toxic overload. And, as I'll reveal in later chapters of this book, many toxic chemicals are specifically engineered to resist breakdown. Although civilized products and comforts have their upsides, toxins from a range of sources are their unacknowledged, nearly invisible downside. Toxic overload may consist of any or all of the following:

1. Industrial toxins, such as heavy metals, pollution, and radiation released by industrial activities

2. Agricultural toxins, such as pesticides, hormones, and herbicides

3. Household toxins from building materials, rugs, paint, and cleaning supplies

4. Toxins in personal care products, including health and beauty aids (HABAs), perfumes, and cosmetics

5. Food toxins, like genetically modified organisms (GMOs), food coloring, artificial flavors, and artificial sweeteners

6. Other consumer-product toxins, such as flame retardants in
children's clothing, toys, and blankets; sealants in cookware,
and more

While we take many of these types of products and services for
granted, the substances they contain (or generate) can harm our bodies
in numerous ways. (See table 1.1.)

Fortunately, not every toxin is harmful to every bodily organ or system. Toxic effects can be major or minor.

Table 1.1. **General Types of Toxicity and Symptoms**

CATEGORY	SYSTEM AFFECTED	COMMON SYMPTOMS
Respiratory	Nose, throat, lungs	Irritation, coughing, choking, tight chest
Gastrointestinal	Stomach, intestines	Nausea, vomiting, diarrhea
Renal	Kidney	Back pain, urinating more or less than usual
Neurological	Brain, spinal cord	Headache, dizziness, confusion, depression, coma, convulsions, memory loss
Hematological	Blood	Anemia (tiredness, weakness), frequent infections
Dermatological	Skin, eyes	Rashes, itching, redness, swelling
Reproductive	Ovaries, testes, fetus	Infertility, miscarriage, menstrual cycle disruption

Many diseases once rare are now epidemic in people of all ages for
reasons doctors can't explain—unless we consider toxins. Take diabetes, which affected only 1 percent of the population sixty years ago:
it is now diagnosed in 10 percent of the population and is expected
to afflict more than 30 percent of all Americans. We are seeing the
rise of cardiovascular disease and obesity in twenty-year-olds, and it is
now commonplace for men and women to suffer from all the ailments

Table 1.1 source: Modified from http://pmep.cce.cornell.edu/profiles/extoxnet/TIB/manifestations.html.

related to aging ten, twenty, or even thirty years earlier than they should. For too many people, forty can feel like fifty or sixty. As you will learn from reading this book, toxins have become the driving factor behind this phenomenon.

In 2010, the President's National Cancer Panel found that "approximately 1.5 million American men, women, and children were diagnosed with cancer, and 562,000 died from the disease. With the growing body of evidence linking environmental exposures to cancer, the public is becoming increasingly aware of the unacceptable burden of cancer resulting from environmental and occupational exposures that could have been prevented."[2]

Unfortunately, since 2010, when the panel presented its findings, there has been no action taken on its recommendations, which included more research into and solid regulation of toxic chemicals.

As a result, since that time toxicity has progressively increased, and most people have no idea how serious this problem has become. It is not just cancer: all chronic disease is caused or aggravated by the pervasive toxins. Don't wait until you have a serious condition like cancer before you take control.

How I Came to Write This Book

The concept that toxins absorbed into our bodies affect human health is not new. Through clinical work with thousands of grateful people, courageous medical pioneers like Rachel Carson, PhD; Bill Rey, MD; Hal Huggins, DDS; Walter Crinnion, ND; and many others have discovered that, while toxic load is a huge problem, we can do something about it. I'm glad I could play a part in these discoveries and in teaching doctors how to detoxify their patients.

Over the almost half century I've been taking care of patients, I've seen a relentless increase in chronic disease, along with a dramatic change in the underlying reasons people are becoming chronically unwell. Like many doctors, I at first didn't fully appreciate the need to promote bodily detoxification. But I became a convert early on, and I've seen smart detox support—which I will offer in *The Toxin Solution*—change lives.

It was by accident that I first found out about, studied, and eventually began to practice detoxification therapy. In 1970, I decided to leave graduate school to go into medical research. Moving from upstate New York to Seattle, I began to work as a research assistant in the Department of Rheumatology at the University of Washington School of Medicine. I loved the laboratory and occasional clinical work and soon decided to pursue a PhD in the field. But then something unexpected happened.

Like many research labs around the world, our lab sought a cure for the various forms of arthritis. When the fiancée of my college roommate told me that her supposedly "incurable" juvenile arthritis was now cured, I was amazed and asked her how this happened.

"I went to a naturopathic doctor," she told me.

My response was "Huh?"

Looking back, I was pretty naive about medicine: I didn't know there were any other healing arts, not even chiropractic.

Being naturally quite inquisitive and scientifically oriented, I went to this naturopathic doctor and asked what he did for my friend. His response? "I detoxified her liver, taught her how to eat, and gave her some vitamins." Another "Huh?" from me. What did her liver have to do with her hands and knees being swollen? I then asked if I could spend a few days watching him see patients. I saw case after case of "incurable" patients being helped by this wonderful healer through what seemed much simpler, far safer, and more sensible "natural" interventions. I was hooked, and to my good fortune, the last naturopathic medicine school in all of North America was in Seattle. Yes, the AMA had won every battle and greatly diminished the profession—but they didn't quite win the war. As my beloved Dr. John Bastyr told us as students, paraphrasing Shakespeare, "No matter the obstacles they place, the truth of our medicine will out."

As a naturopathic medical student in the early 1970s, I learned about toxicity and detoxification. Although we were taught some great detoxification protocols, at the time there was no scientific validation for them. The mechanisms of toxicity and protocols for detoxification were simply unknown. So, while I was aware of the principle of detox, it didn't affect my clinical thinking very much. Then, in about my sixth month of practice, two patients transformed my understanding.

Peter's and Don's Stories

Peter came to my office because of his leukemia. He appeared to have been effectively treated with chemotherapy, but he wondered why, at age thirty, he had developed this cancer. I learned that he ate like everyone else (poorly) and didn't take any vitamins. He did get a lot of exercise, since he worked on a farm. A physical exam revealed nothing unusual for a young man his age, and a screening lab test found no abnormalities. (I wish I could go back to look at those old lab tests with the knowledge I have now.) All I could offer him at the time was the advice to simply clean up his diet and take a good-quality multivitamin and mineral.

Then, two weeks later, Don came to my office with essentially the same presentation. He also worked on a farm. Hmm, I wondered, could there be a connection between their illness and their exposure to chemical fertilizers, pesticides, and herbicides? At my request, both brought me the labels from the drums that contained the products they were using on the farms.

I consulted a toxicology textbook to learn about the chemicals these two men had been spraying on the fields. I dug into the relevant chapters, and lo and behold, I found that farmers in general were showing a significantly increased risk of most blood cancers, apparently in proportion to their use of modern farm chemicals. I gulped a bit, spent $150 (a lot of money for a struggling young practitioner in an unpopular field of medicine) to buy the textbook, and started reading.

Tracking the connections between supposedly benign chemicals and human health opened my eyes. It became the work of a lifetime. In *The Toxin Solution,* I hope to open your eyes. A lot of people prefer not to know about the toxin–health connection, because it's just too scary and requires change. But knowing gives you two options that you lack when you just take our toxic world for granted. Once you know, you have a new opportunity to:

1. Make dietary and lifestyle choices to lessen the toxins you absorb.
2. Undergo the Toxin Solution on a regular basis to release your toxic load.

Our Toxic World

Toxins enter our bodies every day through the food we eat, the water we drink, the air we breathe, the substances we touch or apply to our faces and bodies—even through the drugs and treatments prescribed by doctors and dentists. Until you reflect upon all that you take in without a second thought, the many ways you are exposed to toxins may seem hidden and surprising.

For example, do you ever order out for pizza? To increase their durability and confer heat resistance, pizza boxes are widely treated with perfluorinated alkylated substances (PFASs) to make them resistant to water and to grease stains. PFASs cause low-dose endocrine disruption and immunotoxicity.[3] In other words, exposure to them can either suppress or imbalance the immune system, increasing risk of infection and autoimmune conditions. PFASs are used on a wide range of other products, including nonstick cooking pans and utensils, "breathable" rain gear, stain-resistant sprays for furniture, sleeping bags, electronics (cell phones and hard disk drives), backpacks, footwear, and even hospital equipment. They can be found in the needles, pacemakers, stents, hospital gowns, and even the divider curtains used in hospitals.

A hazardous substance moves into the human body via what scientists call "an exposure pathway." Unfortunately, as a study published in 2015 notes, breast-feeding is an important exposure pathway for PFASs.[4] The greater the frequency of breast-feeding, the higher the concentrations of PFASs in infants and babies studied at ages eleven months, eighteen months, and five years.[5] What people use, handle, contact, inhale, smell, or eat is absorbed into their bodies and even passed along to the next generation. How sad that newborns (and, as we will see later, even infants in utero) are absorbing the toxic chemicals that flood our world.

How did we come to this?

Over the last seventy-five years, chemistry has brought Americans and others in the "civilized" world a wide range of useful products and services that most of us take for granted. In becoming dependent on everything from fast food to heating fuel to commercially produced baby blankets, we've made certain assumptions. Most of us have assumed either that all these wonders are "inert"—that is, that they are biologically inactive, with no discernible impact on biology and living things—or that it is safe to overlook their chemical effects as insignificant. Yet over fifty years ago, pioneering ecologist Rachel Carson cautioned about chemicals in our food in her breakthrough book *Silent Spring.* "A Who's Who of pesticides," she wrote, is "of concern to us all. If we are going to live so intimately with these chemicals, eating and drinking them, taking them into the very marrow of our bones—we had better know something about their nature and their power."[6]

The unfortunate reality is that half a century later, we still have much to learn, and the toxin problem has become much, much worse. The President's Cancer Panel of 2010 found that "with nearly 80,000 chemicals on the market in the United States, many of which are used by millions of Americans in their daily lives and are un- or understudied and largely unregulated, exposure to potential environmental carcinogens is widespread."[7]

Dr. Sanjay Gupta, a practicing neurosurgeon and CNN's chief medical correspondent, notes that "up to 200 chemicals are in the blood of babies before they're even born. The exact ramifications of the presence of all these chemicals is unclear. Certainly, we have seen an increase in various diseases, from asthma and autism to childhood obesity. It will take a national long-term study to say for sure what these chemicals may be contributing."[8]

"Only a few hundred of the more than 80,000 chemicals in use in the United States have been tested for safety," writes Nicholas Kristof of the *New York Times,* quoting the President's Cancer Panel: "Many known or suspected carcinogens are completely unregulated."[9]

While concerned people work hard to avoid individual exposure, Ansje Miller, the coauthor of a 2013 report released by the Center for the Environment and Health, notes that "many harmful chemicals that we have been working so hard to eliminate from consumer products are now being used"[10] in industrial activities such as hydraulic fracturing (hydrofracking).

Large-scale exposures to pollutants where you live is becoming increasingly impossible to avoid. A University of Pittsburgh study published in 2015 found that "living close to a high number of 'fracked' natural gas wells may be linked to an increased risk of having a lower-birth-weight baby."[11] This may be due in part to heavy metals, radiation, and carcinogens used in (or released by) drilling for unconventional sources of gas.

You may not live near fracking wells, but few communities are immune to pollutants of one kind or another. For example, if you live in New England, you likely have elevated mercury levels from the burning of contaminated coal for electricity generation. Or you may have high levels of arsenic if you're one of the 10 percent of Americans drinking from commercial water supplies. In fact, a 2000 study showed that as many as fifty-six million Americans had unsafe levels of arsenic in their water—and that was only in the twenty-five states that were studied.[12] Or you may go to work every day unaware of the harmful chemicals in your workplace. One study out of Harvard determined that Americans have collectively forfeited 41 million IQ points as a result of exposure to lead, mercury, and organophosphate pesticides.[13]

The bottom line is that if you are like most people, your body is storing many of the toxins I cover in this book. It is storing them wherever it can—in your bones, in your brain, in your blood, and in your fat. You don't want them there. But you will never release these toxins from your body until your detox system is itself detoxified and doing a first-rate job of getting those toxins out.

Jack's Story

Jack was a wooden-boat builder in Port Townsend, Washington. In my region, the Pacific Northwest, many boat builders are routinely exposed to harmful chemicals from the paints and fiberglass products used to protect the hulls of boats.

Although still a relatively young man, Jack had become progressively debilitated. He felt tired all the time and had no energy to devote to his family. For unknown reasons, his symptoms worsened in the winter. By the time he came to see me, he had become so weak he was hardly able to get out of bed in the morning. Like many people who consult me, he had already seen several medical doctors. Unable to pinpoint any recognizable disease, they had no treatment to offer him. Jack told me he felt as if he had the flu all the time. He was desperate for answers, since he had a wife and young children to support. Fortunately, a bit of detective work quickly pinpointed the cause of his problems.

The special paints used on boat hulls contain varnishes to preserve the wood and heavy metals to keep barnacles from growing on boat bottoms. Although Jack was somewhat able to tolerate these toxins in the summer, to keep his workshop warm in the winter he closed all the doors and windows. Despite the vents, the higher concentration of toxins delivered an increased exposure when he breathed in the polluted air or forgot to wear gloves to prevent topical absorption. Since the Occupational

Safety and Health Administration (OSHA—which regulates workplace safety) had approved his workplace, Jack assumed that the chemicals he worked with were perfectly safe. He rarely wore a protective mask. To make matters worse, his living space was right next door to his workshop and smelled of solvents!

Jack had an enlarged and very sensitive liver. His hands were discolored, and his complexion appeared waxen. I immediately put him on an intensive detoxification program. He stopped working for one week and moved his family several blocks away to avoid exposure while he began to detox.

To stimulate his detoxification processes, Jack went on a one-week modified food fast, emphasizing raw and cooked fruits and vegetables—the very same diet you will be following in this book. (See chapter 3.) He also took the same supplements I will recommend in chapter 5 for detoxing the liver, as well as extra fiber to get the toxins released by the liver bound into his stools.

Jack had a good constitution and responded rapidly to the Toxin Solution. Within a few weeks he was back to his normal, energetic self. Once he returned to work, he installed a heater, opened all the doors and windows in the workshop, and began using gloves and a chemical mask while he worked. By improving the ventilation, rigorously limiting contact exposure, and strongly supporting his detoxification systems, Jack's health and energy were fully restored, giving him ample stamina for fun family activities with his wife and kids, as well as building his beautiful wooden boats.

When I first began treating detox, most people had never heard of the concept. How things have changed! Now, it's extremely common for well-informed people to actively seek out detox approaches. And it's due to growing public concern about the mounting toxic load that contributes to symptoms and illness. I applaud this development! But knowing that detox is necessary is not the same thing as fully understanding *how* to safely detox. Nor does it mean that any and all detox approaches are equally effective. For one thing, stirring up a load of toxins and allowing them to circulate in your system isn't a good approach. You must control and manage your detox. To do that, it's essential that the organs of elimination themselves (gut, liver, and kidneys) first be repaired. And to ensure that you initiate detox safely, those organs must be repaired in the right sequence. Otherwise, you can unleash more toxins than your body can safely handle. Yes, you need to detox, but your body's detoxification organs need help first—a lot of help—to detox effectively. And that's what the Toxin Solution will provide.

The problem is that, since conventional medicine is largely ignorant about detoxification, when it comes to using a truly science-based approach, people have almost no guidance.

Why Has It Taken So Long to Recognize the Problem with Toxins?

You may be wondering, *If this is such a big problem, why don't you hear more about it?* There are several reasons—all due to shortfalls in conventional medicine and its research agenda.

Conventional medicine works great where there is a simple connection between the cause of a disease, like an infecting organism, and the treatment, like an antibiotic. However, this model fails in many areas— for example, when a disease has multiple causes or when single causes are associated with multiple diseases.

This model also wrongly assumes that people are standard. On the contrary, each of us is biochemically unique—especially in our ability to detoxify the huge range of poisons we are exposed to. This really shows up with toxicity: some people may be very good at getting rid of specific toxins— like smokers who live to over a hundred without lung cancer—while for most of us, ridding the body of toxins isn't easy. Conventional medicine doesn't measure toxic levels (except in those who have had obvious workplace exposure) and pays no attention to detox capacity. It's easy to dismiss the need for detoxification when you don't assess these markers. But where does that leave you? Outside of obvious high-level toxic exposures—like those that occur in specific jobs or in industrial accidents or spills—doctors can rarely point to one toxin as the cause of disease onset.

Conventional medicine spends its big research bucks on devising new pharmaceutical medications, not on investigating what makes people sick to begin with. In addition, as crass as this sounds, there is no one who commercially benefits from finding these toxin connections, so the research dollars are scarce. As a result, until quite recently researchers have been hamstrung in their efforts to adequately assess the many problems of toxicity.

How Chemical Toxins Dysregulate Your Body

So how exactly do toxins produce all of these different kinds of health issues and symptoms? And why is the range of problems so diverse? According to the Pesticide Information Project of Cooperative Extension Offices of Cornell University, Michigan State University, Oregon State University, and University of California at Davis,[14] when a chemical toxin enters your body, it actually alters the speed at which many key functions take place. This alteration can decrease the activity of the enzymes that are required for every bodily function. For example, toxins may:

- Increase or decrease heart rate.
- Interrupt neuron connections necessary for the brain to function.
- Decrease the production of thyroid hormones that regulate how fast enzymes work.
- Block insulin-receptor sites on cells so sugar can't get in to produce energy.

Obviously, when extreme, these effects can even be life-threatening. Any toxic exposure, whether it is chronic (over a long period) or acute (a sudden high exposure), starts with biochemical changes. These in turn affect the cells' function. The activity—or dysfunction—determines how well the organs and systems work. Any given toxin may have very broad effects or cause only a very limited change in a particular organ or area. It depends on the toxin, the dosage, and each person's unique DNA.

For example, if someone ingests an insecticide such as parathion, it can inactivate an enzyme that affects communication between nerves. At the cellular level, this produces changes that lead to sweating. But that is not the sole effect.

Since that enzyme works throughout the body, its inactivation produces widespread physiological changes. These include reproductive, nervous-system, and possibly carcinogenic effects.[15]

How Toxins Cause Disease

Although the word *toxin* sounds scary, most people don't grasp precisely how toxins interact with human physiology and how long this has been a problem for humans. Doctors noticed almost two hundred years ago that toxins like mercury were causing "mad hatter disease." It was also known that toxicity from leaded water pipes was a major cause of the decline of the Roman Empire. But in the past, these toxins were largely limited to occupational exposure. Only people who performed certain specific tasks—coal miners, who inhale coal dust, for example—were known to be casualties. Doctors didn't consider the rest of the population to be at risk. But with the explosion of industrial activity and products, that has changed. Following more research, scientists and perceptive clinicians now better understand that toxicity affects most—if not all—of the population. The more research I look at and the more patients I care for, the more convinced I am that we are seeing only the tip of the iceberg.

Basically, there are eight ways toxins damage our bodies:

1. **Toxins poison enzymes** so they don't work properly. Our bodies are enzyme engines. Every physiological function depends on enzymes to manufacture molecules, produce energy, and create

cell structures. Toxins damage enzymes and thus undermine countless bodily functions—inhibiting the production of hemoglobin in the blood, for example, or lowering the body's capacity to prevent the free-radical damage that accelerates aging.

2. **Toxins displace structural minerals,** resulting in weaker bones. People need to maintain healthy bone mass for lifelong mobility. When toxins displace the calcium present in bone, there is a twofold effect: weaker skeletal structures and increased toxins, released by bone loss, which circulate throughout the body.

3. **Toxins damage the organs.** Toxins damage nearly all your organs and systems. The Toxin Solution will focus specifically on the detox organs. If your digestive tract, liver, and kidneys are so toxic they are unable to detox effectively, your detoxification will backfire, and your body will remain toxic.

4. **Toxins damage DNA,** which increases the rate of aging and degeneration. Many commonly used pesticides, phthalates, improperly detoxified estrogens, and products containing benzene damage DNA.

5. **Toxins modify gene expression.** Our genes switch off and on to adapt to changes in our bodies and the outer environment. But many toxins activate or suppress our genes in undesirable ways. The results are not only individual health problems but also effects that span generations.

6. **Toxins damage cell membranes** so they don't respond properly. "Signaling" in the body happens in the cell membranes. Damage to these membranes prevents them from getting important messages—insulin not signaling the cells to absorb more sugar, for example, or muscle cells not responding to the message from magnesium to relax.

7. **Toxins interfere with hormones** and cause imbalances. Toxins induce, inhibit, mimic, and block hormones. One example: Arsenic disrupts thyroid hormone receptors on the cells, so the

cells don't get the message from the thyroid hormones that cause them to rev up metabolism. The result is inexplicable fatigue. (I'll present more examples in chapter 2.)

8. Last but not least, **toxins actually impair your ability to detoxify**—and this is the worst problem of all.

When you are very toxic and desperately need to detoxify, it's harder to do than when you are *not* toxic. In other words, just when you need your detox systems most (to address health issues), your hard-working detox system is most likely to be functioning below par. Why? Because the heavy toxic load you already carry has overwhelmed your detox capacity. That's right. The more toxins you have burdening your body, the greater the damage to your body's detoxification pathways.

That's why the Toxin Solution comprehensively addresses the biggest challenge—restoring your detox organs, and with them your detox pathways. The net result is that you then can readily release toxins from your body.

The Risks of Mercury Exposure

Let's take a closer look at one extremely harmful heavy metal. When present in the body, mercury, a well-established neurotoxin, poisons the nervous system. Suffice it to say here that when your brain and nervous system don't function right, nothing is going to go right. Fatigue—a key reason many patients see doctors—is the foremost symptom, affecting over a quarter of those with too much mercury.

Where does that mercury come from, and where does it go? Table 1.2 shows the primary sources of mercury, apart from occupational and industrial exposures.

Amalgams, also called "silver fillings," are typically 55 percent mercury. Each filling releases about 1 μg (one microgram) of mercury *every* day, and since the average adult in North America has ten fillings, that means 10 μg every day. Is that mercury absorbed into your body? Yes, which is why it shows up in the urine in proportion to the amount of mercury in a person's mouth.

Table 1.2. **Primary Sources of Mercury, in Micrograms per Day (μg /d)**

SOURCE	TYPICAL DOSAGE
Amalgams	10 μg /d
Fish	2.3 μg /d
Water	0.3 μg /d
Air	Variable according to location
Vaccinations	Variable according to vaccine

To make matters worse, the half-life of mercury is two months. The half-life measures how long it takes for 50 percent of a substance to be cleared from the body. As you can see in table 1.3, many toxic metals and chemicals that get into our bodies have half-lives measured in months and years! This means they are extremely difficult to get rid of.

Table 1.3. **Half-Lives of Typical Toxins in the Blood**

TOXIN	HALF-LIFE
Arsenic	2–4 days (CDC)
Benzene	0.5–1 day
Cadmium	16 years
Chlordane	3–4 days
DDT	6–10 years
Dieldrin	2–12 months
Ethanol	15 percent/hour
Lead	1–1.5 months (2–30 years in bone)
Mercury	2 months (CDC)
PCBs	2–30 years!
Toluene	0.5–3 days

Table 1.2 source: M. J. Vimy and F. L. Lorscheider, "Dental amalgam mercury daily dose estimated from intra-oral vapor measurements: A predictor of mercury accumulation in human tissues," *Journal of Trace Elements in Experimental Medicine* 3 (1990): 111–23.

Table 1.3 source: M. Schulz, S. Iwersen-Bergmann, H. Andresen, and A. Schmoldt, "Therapeutic and toxic blood concentrations of nearly 1,000 drugs and other xenobiotics," *Critical Care* 16, no. 4 (2012): R136.

Unfortunately, the data get worse. Mercury in pregnant and nursing women gets into the fetus. It actually reaches higher levels in the fetus, with the fetal brain containing levels 40 percent higher than the mother's brain—a disaster for a developing neurological system. And where does that mercury mostly come from? The mother's fillings.[16] Sadly, mercury in breast milk also ends up in the infant. Mothers-to-be, one of the best gifts you can give your future child is to get the toxins out before you become pregnant.

Now, let's see exactly how toxic mercury load undermines detox capacity. When doctors examine brain mercury levels in someone with a mouthful of mercury amalgam fillings, they find that these levels are disproportionately higher after twelve or more fillings in the mouth. Why? Because mercury transport out of the brain is *slowed* as the blood–brain membrane becomes saturated.[17] In other words, we have a limited capacity to get mercury out of the brain, and once that capacity is used up, the rest of the mercury can't get out. Obviously, you don't want excess mercury stuck in your brain.

This is a good example of how nearly any toxin impairs the body's detox capacities. When the toxic load increases past a certain point, detoxing gets harder. Trust me, you don't want to reach that point. The problem is that, apart from symptoms and disease, you don't know your current toxic load, because conventional medicine mostly ignores toxins, toxic load, and detoxification.

What We Should Be Doing

What do we need to do to gain a complete scientific grasp of how toxins affect health? All of the following.

Track All Toxic Exposures

Despite the need to know the health effects of *all* toxic exposures, from the minor ones to cases of extreme exposure, most research focuses either on acute poisoning or chronic buildup from long-term occupational industrial exposure. The first toxicology textbook I read asserted the widely held view at the time that even though exposure to pesticides and herbicides caused health problems for farmworkers, consumers eating foods grown with those very same agricultural toxins should not be alarmed. Supposedly, their exposure was too low to be a problem.

That seemed to be true—because back then most research covered only a few years of exposure to just one toxin. But what about the reality: decades of exposure to multiple toxins? What about genetic susceptibility? Or nutrient deficiencies that impair the function of detoxification enzymes? Forty years ago, I began to ask those questions. Because I knew what to look for, I soon realized that I could see how toxins were damaging my most susceptible or most exposed patients—the so-called yellow canaries. (This term comes from coal mining—miners used to keep these birds with them in the mines because they were very sensitive to carbon monoxide. The miners knew there was a problem as soon as the birds started to faint.) It has only gotten worse, to the point that these days everyone is affected. What is now called "normal" is a population heavily exposed to toxins.

About ten years ago, researchers finally started asking the right questions and measuring the right parameters. Despite continued resistance from conventional medicine and from agribusiness (and the politicians who accept their campaign donations), these courageous researchers are now clearly documenting the huge health impacts of so many different toxins.

Conduct More Long-Term Research

Almost all the studies focus on high levels of exposure, with little research on low- and medium-level exposure over a long period of time. The good news is that this latter research is finally being done. The bad news is that what is being found is far worse than almost anyone expected.

Identify Individual Variations in Susceptibility to Toxins

One of the big challenges in tracing the connection between your toxic load and your health symptoms is that we each are physiologically unique. As a result, each of us will have a somewhat different pattern of symptoms associated with specific toxins. For example, in the liver, a major detox organ, there can be as much as a thousandfold variation among individuals in the functionality of certain detox enzymes. This is what is happening backstage in the body when one person can better tolerate a given substance than another person with different genetics.

Some people are more susceptible to damage to their immune system, so they will have more allergies and autoimmune problems. For others, their mitochondria might be more susceptible to toxins, so they will become more fatigued. Nonetheless, if you are in less than perfect health, in reading this book you will begin to recognize the toxins whose symptom patterns best match yours. Just don't expect an exact match, and don't expect it to be as simple as one toxin equals one symptom.

Account for Synergistic Effects

Researchers work really hard to isolate single factors so they can be studied. It's a good beginning, but we need to go further, since no one is exposed to just one toxin. Nor does isolating a single toxin capture the breadth of the average person's toxic load. And what about when toxins act together? Those interactions can magnify the damage. They may:

- Cause damage by the same mechanisms.

- Increase the risk of the same disease by different mechanisms.

- Work synergistically to cause more damage than one toxin alone would.

- Use up the body's stores of glutathione—the main molecule that protects us from the oxidative damage caused by toxins.

For example, organochlorine pesticides poison insulin-receptor sites to worsen metabolic syndrome and diabetes.[18] But the effect is worse when the person is also exposed to arsenic, which impairs the ability of the pancreas to secrete insulin.[19] Now you have two different toxic agents attacking the body's ability to regulate blood sugar, each in a different way. The end result after years of exposure is diabetes.

Figure 1.2 shows what happens when a pesticide and aluminum act together on the body to increase disease risk.

Figure 1.2. **Synergistic interaction of pesticides and aluminum**

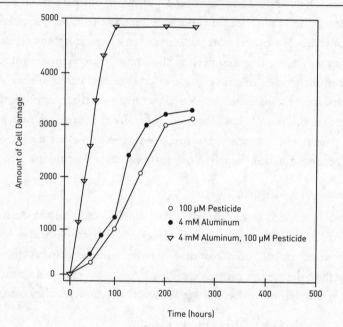

Figure 1.2 incorporates a great deal of research and is just the beginning of the type of assessment necessary to track how toxins contribute to the rising rates of disease. But the bottom line is that no one is exposed to just one single toxin. We are all exposed to many different toxins over time. Some are released fairly rapidly, but some linger in our bodies. And

Figure 1.2 source: V. N. Uversky, J. Li, K. Bower, and A. L. Fink, "Synergistic effects of pesticides and metals on the fibrillation of alpha-synuclein: Implications for Parkinson's disease," *Neurotoxicology* 23, nos. 4–5 (2002): 527–36.

that is why each of us carries a toxic brew within. The goal of this book is to help you reduce the total amount of that brew and lower the levels of the more dangerous toxins.

You may be wondering how big a problem toxicity really is and maybe even thinking it does not apply to you. If you are reading this book, I suspect you are not a smoker, as everyone knows smoking is really bad for us and greatly increases the risk of lung cancer. What would you think if I told you that certain toxins increase the risk of their corresponding diseases to the same degree as smoking cigarettes? Smoking cigarettes doubles your risk of lung cancer. As you can see below, almost everyone has levels of toxins that double the risk of many diseases. After looking at a large amount of research, I think we can now say that toxins are a much *worse* public health problem than smoking, as only 17.9 percent of people in the USA smoke[20] but far more have elevated disease-causing toxin levels.

Table 1.4. **Percent of Population with Doubled Risk of Disease due to Specific Toxins**

TOXIN	DISEASE	% OF POPULATION WITH DOUBLED RISK
PAHs	Asthma	94
PCB 187	Breast cancer	60
Phthalates	Diabetes	55
Lead	ALS (amyotrophic lateral sclerosis)	33
DDT	ADHD (attention deficit hyperactivity disorder)	25
PCBs	Diabetes	25
Dioxin-like PCBs	Rheumatoid arthritis	25
Arsenic	Gout	23
BPA	Diabetes	22
Cigarette smoking	**Lung cancer**	**21**
Arsenic	Diabetes	20
PAHs	Diabetes	20

Table 1.4 source: Data from http://www.cdc.gov/tobacco/data_statistics/fact_sheets/adult_data/cig_smoking.

Even though the connections between toxins and diseases have yet to be studied comprehensively, the results from the latest research reveal that doctors need to account for all toxins—and so do you! You need to be mindful of the toxins you absorb from the foods you eat, the products you use, the water you drink, the air you breathe, and the places where you live and work. The relationship between toxin exposure and disease is far more powerful than any other known disease risk factor.

To understand how toxins interplay with—and worsen—other risk factors, let's take a look at the role of toxins in diabetes.

What Caused the Diabetes Epidemic: Sugar or Toxins?

When I first started my work in health, diabetes was rare. In clinical practice in the late 1970s, every year I would see only a few patients with either type 1 or type 2 diabetes. Diabetes has now become one of the most common diseases seen by doctors every day. As of 2012, the annual costs of diagnosed type 2 diabetes were $245 billion, a 41 percent increase over just five years (from 2007).[21] This gives you an idea of both the price tag and accelerating speed of this epidemic.

Figure 1.3. **The type 2 diabetes epidemic: Percentage of U.S. population with diagnosed diabetes, 1958–2009**

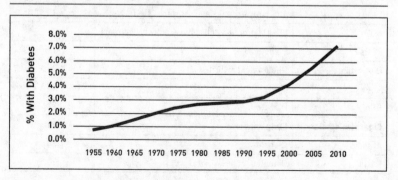

Figure 1.3 source: CDC's Division of Diabetes Translation, National Diabetes Surveillance System, available at http://www.cdc.gov/diabetes/statistics.

Please note that the data in figure 1.3 use the same diagnostic criteria throughout the whole fifty-one-year time period covered by the graph. (Those criteria were changed in 2013, resulting in an even greater number of people now being diagnosed as diabetic.)

Reading this, you might think, *Of course diabetes is more common now. People eat a lot more sugar than in the past!* When you look at sugar consumption over the past two hundred years, though (see figure 1.4), the surprising finding is that while excessive sugar consumption by individuals does correlate with diabetes to some extent, the increase in diabetes didn't start with the consumption of sugar. Then what was going on?

Figure 1.4. **Increasing sugar consumption, 1822–2005**

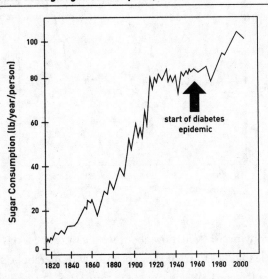

Now take a look at the growing production of chemicals for industrial, personal, and agricultural use. (See figure 1.5.) Wow, an incredibly strong correlation! Of course, we all know that correlation does not prove causation. However, in this instance we have both correlation

Figure 1.4 source: http://wholehealthsource.blogspot.com/2012/02/by-2606-us-diet-will-be-100-percent.html.

and the key mechanisms that explain why and how increased exposure to chemical pollutants could produce (or significantly contribute to) diabetes: *Many chemical pollutants poison insulin-receptor sites on our cells.* These are sites that need to be well functioning so insulin can get sugar into our cells for energy production and protect us from diabetes.

Figure 1.5. **The correlation between chemical production and type 2 diabetes**

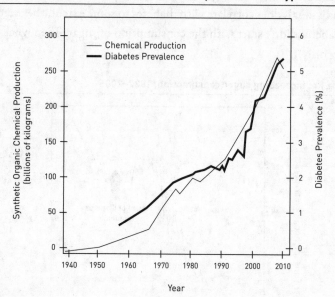

Still not convinced? Well, how about we measure the levels of chemicals in people's bodies to see if they correlate with metabolic syndrome (basically, prediabetes). As you can see in figure 1.6, not only does each of these correlate with prediabetes, but they are synergistic.

Researchers are now finding such a strong connection between these chemicals on the one hand and diabetes and obesity on the other that they are being called *diabetogens* and *obesogens*.

Figure 1.5 source: Brian A. Neel and Robert M. Sargis, "The paradox of progress: Environmental disruption of metabolism and the diabetes epidemic," *Diabetes* 60, no. 7 (2011): 1838–48.

Figure 1.6. **Toxin levels correlate strongly with metabolic syndrome**

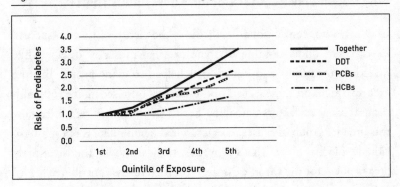

Obviously, this is just one example of how toxins increase your chances of getting one disease. But diabetes is not the sole disease that toxins contribute to.

If you still are not convinced, take a look at how the levels of toxic chemicals in the body correlate with full-blown diabetes risk. As can be seen in figure 1.7, as toxin load goes up, so does the risk of diabetes, with those in the top 10% body load of just one of the many toxins having a worrisome twelvefold increased risk of diabetes!

Figure 1.7. **Toxin levels correlate strongly with diabetes**

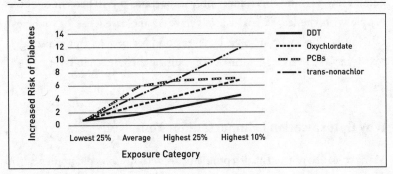

Figure 1.6 source: J. Ukropec, Z. Radikova, M. Huckova, et al., "High prevalence of prediabetes and diabetes in a population exposed to high levels of an organochlorine cocktail," *Diabetologia* 53, no. 5 (2010): 899–906.

Figure 1.7 source: D. H. Lee, I. K. Lee, K. Song, et al., "A strong dose-response relation between serum concentrations of persistent organic pollutants and diabetes: Results from the National Health and Examination Survey 1999–2002," *Diabetes Care* 29, no. 7 (2006): 1638–44.

Why Doesn't My Regular Doctor Know About This?

In many ways, conventional medicine is the victim of its own success. Its excellent understanding of some external causes of disease—like infectious organisms and injury—has helped so many people. But the exclusive focus on these factors blinds doctors from seeing the full, multicausal range of factors damaging health. Nor do they recognize how this broader group of causes interacts with the uniqueness of each individual's biochemistry. That's why the medical model almost entirely breaks down for the chronic diseases to which toxins contribute.

Type 2 diabetes is due to a combination of many possible causes and mechanisms—primarily loss of insulin sensitivity by the cells and impaired ability of the pancreas to secrete insulin. These varied mechanisms are triggered by: obesity,[22] lack of exercise,[23] eating too many refined carbohydrates,[24] a low-fiber diet,[25] too much saturated or hydrogenated fat,[26] and chromium deficiency.[27] To this list we now must add the insulin resistance caused by the many persistent organic pollutants that are building up in our bodies.[28] These are now an even greater risk factor. You will notice that obesity is first on the list above; everyone knows that people who are extremely overweight almost always get diabetes. However, and this is incredibly important, the 10 percent of obese people with the lowest toxin levels have *no* increased risk of diabetes! Obviously, obesity on its own is never good for people. But amazingly, toxins have an even bigger impact on causing diabetes than fat.

Why Detoxification Is Important for You

Many so-called normal health problems are actually *unnecessary* ill health, dysfunction, disease, and deterioration with aging. Research now shows that the allergies, immune impairment, autoimmune disease, degenerative neurological diseases, diabetes, and cancers that have become so common are not normal but are instead due to nutrient deficiencies and an ever-growing toxic load. Even the conventional laboratory tests to detect disease now have "normal" ranges that are not the "healthy" range.

This book contains many case stories showing how to reverse disease by avoiding and eliminating toxins. Many, many people have benefited from this approach.

By understanding the role toxins play in your health—present and future—you can do something about them now by following my comprehensive detox program. Not only will *The Toxin Solution* help to address any current complaints you may have, but, most importantly, it will help to prevent future diseases. I've looked into this topic deeply and am certain that grasping certain basics, and understanding the disease risks that as a society we have foolishly discounted, will motivate you to protect your health.

2

The Causes of Toxic Overload

How Toxins Damage Health and Cause Disease

Throughout *The Toxin Solution*, I speak up as a scientist about the health impacts of chemical exposures. I was a chemistry major in college and intended to enter that field. Like everyone back then, I was entranced by DuPont's "Better Living Through Chemistry," an advertising slogan disseminated in magazines and television well until the 1980s. Once in graduate school, I discovered that chemists' work in labs regularly exposed them to industrial chemicals. Then I read a shocking study that revealed that chemists have a twenty-year shorter than average life span! I realized that if I pursued that career, I was essentially volunteering as a human guinea pig and shortening my life expectancy. My response was: *No, thanks!* And yet in a certain sense we all are part of a giant experiment. Is the human organism able to adapt rapidly enough to carry ever increasing loads of toxins without compromising health? So far, the answer is no. Yet science is just beginning to reveal the health impacts of exposure to this vast soup of toxins.

It's vital to distinguish between avoidable and unavoidable toxins. The avoidable ones you will learn to stay away from on this program. In order to deal with the unavoidable ones, it's vital for everyone to periodically repair their detoxification organs and undergo active detox—as you will be doing over the next nine weeks. Don't forget that although many toxins enter your lungs, skin, and stomach uninvited, there are some that you *ask* to come in. Not intentionally, of course. Who among us would knowingly invite tar to enter our lungs? Or welcome phthalates (chemicals added to plastics to keep them soft)—which increase the risk of breast cancer and birth defects—to penetrate the skin? If you understood the consequences, who would want to eat a sweetener that raises the risks of heart disease and diabetes? But when you smoke, or use certain cosmetics, or drink diet soda, you invite these harmful chemicals along for the ride. There is little point in detoxification if you keep putting new toxins back into your body.

Over 6.5 billion pounds of chemicals are released into the air every year. While I can't offer a comprehensive review of all of them, in this chapter, I will focus on the most important chemicals and metals. You will have ample opportunity to acquaint yourself with others throughout this book.

Taken one by one, many chemicals seem relatively harmless, but if they accumulate in your body they can build to a dramatic toxic load that drains away your health and vitality. During the Eight-Week Toxin Solution, you will access the key bodily mechanisms that neutralize and release toxins. Still, I can't emphasize this enough: it's always better if you don't take them into your body to begin with. Remember table 1.3 in chapter 1, which shows how some toxins take years to eliminate: don't let them in! In this chapter, I'll orient you to the ones you can and can't avoid. I will also offer a basic plan to cut down on avoidable toxins, which you can follow while undergoing the Toxin Solution, and perhaps even lifelong. Once you get the full picture, you will understand why I recommend that everyone periodically (or regularly) both reduce his or her toxins and undertake the Toxin Solution. And of course, I do that myself.

This survey will help you become aware of the specific ways that toxins may be entering your body. While it's not possible to calculate how toxic you actually are (without the more sophisticated lab tests I'll discuss in this book's appendix), the Toxic Troubleshooter will help you pay attention to toxic exposures you may have overlooked.

Toxic Troubleshooter: Have You Been Exposed to Toxins?

1. Do you regularly eat processed foods?

2. Do you regularly eat conventionally raised produce, meat, and dairy?

3. Do you eat farm-raised fish?

4. Do you eat large (i.e., mercury-contaminated) fish?

5. Do you consume high-fructose corn syrup?

6. Do you use more than two health and beauty products per day?

7. Do you live in a house that contains lead pipes or copper plumbing soldered with lead (built prior to 1978)?

8. Are your home, home furnishings, or home finishes (like paint and sealants) new and outgassing chemicals?

9. Do you or your family come into contact with flame-resistant clothing or furnishings sprayed with products to prevent stains?

10. Do you live in a house or work in a building that has mold?

11. Do you have mercury amalgam fillings? How many?

12. Are there mercury-emitting coal-using plants or cement manufacturing plants in your region?

13. Are there fracking wells and/or pipelines in your region?

14. Is there a nuclear power plant in your region? Does it have a poor safety record?

15. Are the water and air in your region polluted?
    Go to www.scorecard.org to check out your region
    or to www.thetoxinsolution.com.

16. If you currently have symptoms, when did they first start?

17. What happened to you in the months prior?

18. When did you last feel well?

19. What makes you feel worse?

20. What makes you feel better?

21. What about medications? Did your symptoms begin shortly
    after you started taking a new medication?

Reconstruct a time line between possible exposures and any declines in your well-being. To do this, go to my website (www.thetoxinsolution .com), where I provide two free tools:

1. A questionnaire that includes all these questions (together
   with additional ones), which will help you determine your
   toxic score.

2. A very helpful time-line tool that helps you easily enter, first,
   your toxic exposures, and next, your health challenges, in
   order to see the relationship between them. Figure 2.1 shows
   how this works.

Low-grade toxic load may first become noticeable through minor symptoms that develop over years. Some people will first observe novel symptoms weeks or months after moving to a new home or starting a new job. It can be a real detective story: When did the black mold start in your bathroom? When did you change dry cleaners and notice that your clothes now smell of chemicals? Did you put new carpeting into your home? How about that new kitchen-cleaning product that was advertised so convincingly on television?

Even if you aren't able to figure out all your most immediate toxic

Figure 2.1. **Relationship between toxic exposures and health challenges, by age**

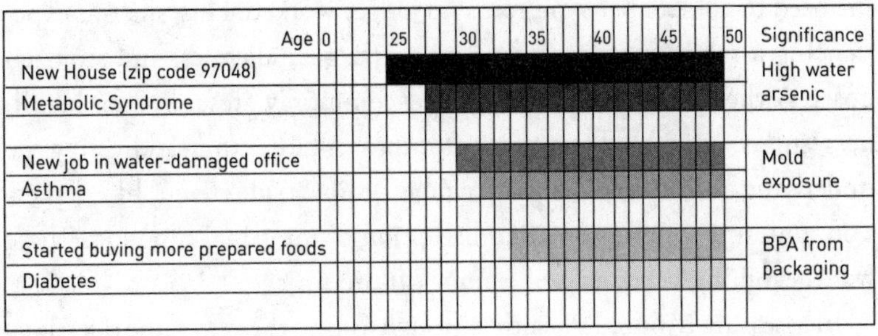

Age	0		25		30		35		40		45		50	Significance
New House (zip code 97048)														High water arsenic
Metabolic Syndrome														
New job in water-damaged office														Mold exposure
Asthma														
Started buying more prepared foods														BPA from packaging
Diabetes														

exposures, by beginning to ask certain questions, you will get on the right track. The first step is noticing toxic sources—both in the past and going forward.

Reducing Your Toxic Load

The two easiest ways to reduce your toxic load starting today are to reduce your consumption of toxin-contaminated foods and your use of toxic health and beauty aids (HABAs). Obviously, you can, and in certain cases must, do a lot more. But unless your health is already seriously undermined, by doing the most basic toxic avoidance and following my program, you will quickly begin to see real health results. Thousands of people, including many who were told they had an "incurable disease," have flocked to my clinic, often as a last resort. Yet once they followed the same protocols you will find in this book and reduced and released their toxins, they felt much healthier and experienced the resolution of a wide range of different diseases.

Mildred's Story

When she came to see me, Mildred had suffered from severe rheumatoid arthritis for thirty years. She was fortunate that there was not much distortion of her joints, but the analgesic and anti-inflammatory drugs she used to control her symptoms no longer worked. Plus, she was experiencing a range of side effects such as fatigue, allergies, and stomach upset. Although the conventional drug commonly prescribed for her illness (sulfasalazine) only suppresses symptoms rather than addressing the underlying causes, such drugs inevitably produce side effects, like depression, immune suppression, and disruption of intestinal function. These were becoming a serious problem for Mildred.

In assessing Mildred's health (through asking the very same questions offered in the Toxic Troubleshooter on page 41 to help you assess your own toxic load), I was able to determine that she had a very high toxic load. In her case, this derived from both the drugs she was taking and a toxic lifestyle. But Mildred had no idea that the foods she ate and the common pesticides and herbicides she used to maintain the bright green lawn and well-cultivated flower garden that surrounded her home were regularly exposing her to an array of chemicals.

Mildred's approach to nutrition was nothing to write home about, either. She regularly consumed (and fed her family) sweetened soft drinks and juices, canned vegetables, soup and gravy mixes, packaged mashed potatoes, and nitrate-loaded meats like hot dogs, along with ample amounts of junk food and candy.

I put her on an earlier version of the nine-week detoxification program I will be guiding you through in this book, and helped her improve her diet. Over two months of the program, her arthritis symptoms improved by 75 percent, and she decreased her use of drugs by over 50 percent. Ironically, at the time I considered myself a failure because I was not able to totally eliminate her arthritis, as total cure was my standard for success, but Mildred saw it quite differently. She was very grateful that I had helped improve her health and decrease her disease burden so much that she was able to lower drug dosages to levels where she no longer experienced those uncomfortable side effects.

What I want you to take way from Mildred's story (along with the many other cases I will share throughout this book) is that what are identified as specific diseases, such as arthritis, diabetes, and heart disease, may all share a similar contributing root cause: toxicity. By reducing the toxin load, you give your body a chance to heal, you can alleviate the disease symptoms, lessen (or eliminate) the disease itself, and reduce your need for drugs that only suppress the symptoms while causing undesirable side effects.

So let's move on to look at some easy ways to reduce your toxic load immediately.

In this chapter, you will first eliminate toxic health and beauty aids. In the next, you will begin the Two-Week Jumpstart Diet, which eliminates toxins in food. If you do nothing else on the program, doing just these two things will make a major difference. Of course, there are other things that I will recommend that you address as well, but these are the basics.

Health and Beauty Aids (HABAs)

Many people slather on lotions and potions to enhance attractiveness, mistakenly assuming that the skin is an impermeable barrier. According to the Collaborative on Health and the Environment, "The average woman in the U.S. uses about 12 personal care and cosmetic products daily. The average man uses about 6."[1] The chemicals they contain easily pass from the skin into the body within minutes of their application. Studies find them in the bloodstream, and in body tissues like the breasts.[2]

Recently, a Missouri jury ordered Johnson & Johnson to pay $72 million to the family of a woman whose death from ovarian cancer was associated with the daily use of talcum-based Johnson's Baby Powder and the company's Shower to Shower products.[3] This is not the first such case.

Most people don't think twice about what the face creams, aftershave, shampoo, antiperspirants, and cosmetics they use on a daily basis actually contain: petroleum by-products, cancer-causing chemicals, and hormonally disruptive fragrances, to name just a few. Although they are widely sold and advertised, seemingly benign personal-care and cosmetic products contain nearly ten thousand untested and unregulated chemicals, according to the Center for Environmental Health (CEH).[4]

You might think that reading the label will tell you everything that is in the product (especially since the list of chemical ingredients is typically very long). But manufacturers aren't required to disclose fragrances or other chemicals that are defined as "trade secrets." Yes, that big loophole allows a lot of toxic exposure without disclosure.

Many chemicals go by innocuous-sounding abbreviations. In table 2.1, I list some of these chemicals, what they are used in, and how they cause problems. This is most definitely *not* a full list. The Environmental Working Group's Skin Deep database contains data on many products with toxic ingredients—as well as healthier options. With the Think Dirty app (www.thinkdirtyapp.com), cocreated by the CEH and the Breast Cancer Fund, you can scan the barcodes of products to determine what they contain. In the next section, I will cover a group of these chemicals with particularly strong disease associations—phthalates.

Table 2.1. **Chemicals Found in Health and Beauty Aids**

CHEMICAL	PURPOSE	TOXICITY EXAMPLE
Acrylates	Artificial nails	Cancer, fetal damage
Aluminum	Antiperspirant	Controversial connection to Alzheimer's disease
Dibutyl phthalate (DBP)	Solvent and preservative for coloring agents and fragrances	Endocrine disruption, diabetes
Diethanolamine (DEA)	Moisturizer	Converted to cancer-causing nitrosamines, skin cancer
Parabens	Preservative and fragrance	Endocrine disruption, breast cancer
Phenylenediamine (CI+number)	Hair dye	Derived from coal tar, resulting in a wide range of toxic contaminants
Quaternium-15, DMDM hydantoin, imidazolidinyl urea, etc.	Preservatives	Release formaldehyde, a known carcinogen
Triclosan	Antimicrobial	Endocrine disruption

Phthalates

Phthalates, which I mentioned earlier, are a family of organic chemicals used to solubilize and stabilize fragrances in cosmetics. They are also used in many other products as plasticizers (to increase flexibility, transparency, and durability). Diethyl phthalate and dibutyl phthalate are especially common in health and beauty aids—except in Europe, where they have now been banned. But if you eat foods that have been packaged or stored in plastic containers, that is also an avenue of significant exposure, because fatty foods like milk, butter, and meats readily absorb these chemicals.

Phthalates are called *endocrine disruptors* because they play havoc with human hormones. They do this by interacting with the endocrine receptor sites located on every cell in your body. In this way they can indiscriminately increase or decrease hormone-mediated cell activities. For example, men who use aftershave, cologne, deodorants, or body washes to make themselves smell "sexy" are actively decreasing testosterone activity and thereby making themselves *less* manly. Although being a man is about more than sexual performance, the very products a man might purchase to supposedly increase his attractiveness could lower his energy and undermine his sexual performance. That's just one example. Here's another—one that's even worse: a recent study of a group of women found that children born to women who had the most phthalates in their bodies have an IQ that is lower by 6.7 points![5] The same study showed that the damage to their intelligence had not resolved by age seven, suggesting that it is permanent.

During the critical time window during which a baby's brain forms the growing and interconnecting neurons that determine brain function and intelligence, children are especially susceptible to toxins. IQ depends on the number of neurons, and even more on the interconnections of the neurons. These are stimulated by a factor known as brain-derived neurotrophic factor. Exposure to phthalates such as those found in nail polish, perfumes, and plastic wrap turns down the activity of the genes that produce this critical brain-development molecule.[6]

Figure 2.2 very effectively shows how HABAs increase phthalates in direct proportion to their use.

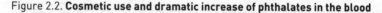

Figure 2.2. **Cosmetic use and dramatic increase of phthalates in the blood**

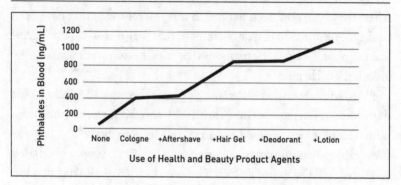

As you can see, a person who uses all the common cosmetics has levels of these poisons in his or her blood about thirty times higher than someone who uses none of them!

Lead

Public health officials removed lead from gasoline and house paint, but they left it in lipstick. Go figure. In 2007, the Campaign for Safe Cosmetics (www.safecosmetics.org) tested thirty-three lipstick brands and found that 61 percent contained lead, with levels ranging up to 0.65 parts per million (ppm). Both drugstore brands and high-end brands (like Dior) contained lead. A follow-up study found lead levels ranging from 0.09 to 3.06 ppm in all lipstick brands studied, with the worst culprits being those produced by Procter & Gamble, Maybelline, and Revlon. Although it may seem that a single application is harmless,

Figure 2.2 source: S. M. Duty, R. M. Ackerman, A. M. Calafat, and R. Hauser, "Personal care product use predicts urinary concentrations of some phthalate monoesters," *Environmental Health Perspectives* 113, no. 11 (2005): 1530–35.

there is no safe exposure level for lead, and there are many sources of everyday exposure. Women apply these products daily over many years. "Unfortunately, nobody is watching the store," notes Stacy Malkan, founder of the Campaign for Safe Cosmetics. "Companies in the U.S. are allowed to put ingredients into personal care products with no required safety testing, and without disclosing all the ingredients."[7]

Sending Your Body a Consistent Message

During the Nine-Week Toxin Solution, you will be asking your body to release toxins. You will get the best results if you don't send your body mixed messages—telling it to release toxins while at the same time continuing to take them in. That is why I invite you to limit your exposure to the toxins in health and beauty aids over the next nine weeks. Here's how.

1. Cut down your daily use of HABAs to one to two products for men and two to three products for women.

2. Read the labels of the products you plan to use, and become aware of what they actually contain.

3. If your must-use products contain questionable ingredients, such as those I list in table 2.1, replace them with healthier ones. You can usually find these at health-food stores, but make sure to read labels. HABAs are not currently regulated. That means that the label "natural" is meaningless. Buying organic products is your safest bet. But you can also find healthy products that aren't necessarily organic by choosing ones with minimal and safe ingredients. For example, coconut oil would not even count as a HABA because it is food grade. It can be used as a face and body moisturizer, a makeup remover, even a hair conditioner. Similarly, an unscented soap made of coconut oil can be used for cleansing, or as a shaving soap.

Nearly every product you use has a safer alternative; you can use the Think Dirty app to find it.

Can cutting down on these products really lower your toxic exposure? Yes, it can. The HERMOSA study[8] helped a group of one hundred Latina students reduce exposure to endocrine disruptors (EDCs) in beauty products. For three days, study participants replaced their usual personal-care products with ones that were free of parabens, phthalates, triclosan, and oxybenzone (used in sunscreen). Measurements of EDC levels in urine before and after the intervention showed much lower levels afterward. Most of the products selected were widely available health-store brands.

Just cutting down on the number of products is a great beginning. Bottom line: decrease toxic exposure whenever you can.

But what about the toxins you can't so easily avoid? Why are they out there? As you will see, though it's possible to eliminate your exposure to lead and phthalates in consumer products, that doesn't mean you're home free.

It's Hard to Avoid Toxins

Have you ever moved to a home or apartment where you had to sign a "lead paint disclosure" form? Since lead is so dangerous, these forms are standard in most residential contracts to ensure that a home purchaser (or renter) does not come back later to sue the seller (or landlord) for lead's damaging health effects. Houses painted with white paint before 1978 have high lead levels. Houses built or remodeled before 1984 often have lead in the pipe solder. Instead of studying and routinely eliminating harmful substances before they reach the public, industries, legislators, and regulatory agencies have it set up so that toxins are put out there until a mass outcry gets them removed. The public health measures that got lead out of gasoline and paint *were* effective: since the ban, levels of lead in human blood have dropped substantially. However, from prior use, lead-based paint and gasoline are still present. Nor were these the sole lead sources. To this day, lead is used in aviation fuel, lipstick, and elsewhere. Although many people, myself included, would like to see the government allow citizens the freedom to make their own choices, it's not possible for us as individuals to simply avoid every toxin out there on our own. This is one place where science and government can work together to keep toxic ingredients out of products (or at least to fully disclose the ingredients). So far, they have not done such a great job of it.

When it comes to a substance so toxic that it is not safe at any level (especially for children), how do we wind up allowing it and calling it safe?

In general, most "safe" levels for toxins are defined as the levels seen in 95 percent of the "normal" population. Since the "normal" population carries a heavy toxic load and suffers poor health and a lot of chronic disease, that is not a healthy baseline. As we've seen, due to the failure to undertake studies, along with chemical-industry lobbying, decades can pass before the regulators figure out how (and have the fortitude) to ban or limit an unsafe substance.

For example, the "safe" blood lead levels (BLLs) used to be 60 μg/dL (micrograms per deciliter) of blood. But researchers found many health problems below that level, so about every decade the regulators kept dropping the "safe" level. With that level now at 10 μg/dL, research still shows an increased incidence of death from all causes—including cardiovascular disease and cancer—in people with lead in the range of 5.0 to 10.0 μg/dL.[9] In other words, scientists try to agree on a benchmark for safety, but some things should be considered unsafe at any level. Because they are. (In figure 2.3, the open dots are the level considered safe and the filled dots are the average level in the population.)

In July 2012, the Centers for Disease Control and Prevention (CDC) determined that lead in the range of 10.0 to 5.0 μg/dL is highly problematic for children. Does that mean that children beneath the lowest end of BLLs are safe? No. Children who have whole-blood lead concentrations of less than 5 μg/dL (supposedly safe) have a measurably lower IQ. Twenty-four million U.S. children have BLLs between 5.0 and 9.9 μg/dL.[10]

Figure 2.3. **"Safe" and average blood lead levels, 1965–2010**

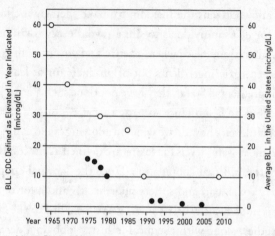

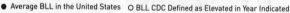

I built my life on what I had the privilege to learn. I built an educational institution to teach others—and to help millions more. What I cover in this book is based on learning, practice, and research. Incapacitating the intelligence of the next generation is no minor matter. Table 2.2 shows the symptoms in children and adults as lead levels increase. What do a selection of the symptoms covered sound like to you?

- Decreased learning and memory

- Decreased verbal ability

- Impaired fine motor coordination

- Low IQ

- Impaired speech and hearing

To me, they describe a coming generation of Americans who at best will have serious learning incapacities. It is not lead alone that damages the brains and the bodies of the unborn and of children.

Figure 2.3 source: http://www.environment.ucla.edu/reportcard/article3772.html, accessed January 10, 2015.

- Phthalates decrease the production of the key molecule in the brain that helps neurons evolve and interconnect.

- Organophosphates (commonly used in agriculture) were developed as neurological poisons for chemical warfare in World War I.

- GMOs were designed to allow excessive use of the weed killer glyphosate, which increases cancer risk.

How did we come to accept the idea that putting these poisons in our food is a good thing?! As discussed elsewhere in this book, not only do these toxins decrease IQ in children; they also double the incidence of ADHD (attention deficit hyperactivity disorder) and behavioral problems.

Table 2.2. **Symptoms as Lead Levels Increase**

LEVEL OF TOXICITY	BLOOD LEAD CONCENTRA-TION (µG/DL)	CLINICAL PRESENTATION	
		CHILDREN	ADULTS
Asymptomatic or impaired abilities	<10	Decreased learning and memory, decreased verbal ability, impaired fine motor coordination, signs of ADHD or hyperactivity, lower IQ, impaired speech and hearing	
Mild	10–39	Myalgia or parasthesia, irritability, mild fatigue/lethargy, occasional abdominal discomfort	
Moderate	>40–50	Arthralgia, difficulty concentrating, general fatigue, headache, muscular exhaustibility, tremor, weight loss, vomiting, constipation, diffuse abdominal pain	Fatigue, somnolence, moodiness, lessened leisure interest, impaired psychometrics, chronic hypertensive effects, reproductive effects
Severe	>70–80	Lead lines (blueish black appearance on gingival tissue), colic (intermittent, severe cramps), parasthesia or paralysis, encephalopathy	Headache, memory loss, decreased libido, insomnia, metallic taste, abdominal pain, constipation, myalgia/arthralgia, nephropathy
Severe, acute	>100–150	Encephalopathy, seizures, anemia, nephropathy	Encephalopathy, various CNS effects, anemia, nephropathy

Table 2.2 source: R. C. Gracia and W. R. Snodgrass, "Lead toxicity and chelation therapy," *American Journal of Health-System Pharmacy* 64, no. 1 (2007): 45–53.

Connie's Story

I don't often treat patients with serious emergencies, so I was surprised to get a call from Connie, who wanted to see me immediately about her sudden loss of vision. I rushed her into my exam room. Connie was a healthy-looking thirty-year-old woman. For the past few days, she had been experiencing progressively greater difficulty reading, and the world was starting to look blurry. That morning, she had experienced sudden complete loss of vision in her right eye, which prompted her call. She also had some pain, which was worse when she moved her eyes, and she was starting to feel tired and weak. As you might expect, she was quite frightened.

Before these symptoms appeared, Connie was healthy. She ate a whole-foods organic diet and exercised regularly. Although the results of my neurological exams were normal, I saw worrisome swelling in the back of her eye and conducted a blood test. I found something seen in only a few diseases (basophilic stippling, for the technically minded), in certain kinds of anemia, and in toxicity from arsenic or lead. Hmm . . . time for some detective work.

I learned that Connie lived on a houseboat at the end of a dock on Lake Union. A new water pipe had recently been installed, and I immediately suspected lead exposure from the solder used. It turned out that Connie loved tea and drank a dozen cups a day.

"Do you empty out the tea kettle every time, or do you simply keep adding water?" I asked. Her answer was the latter. This meant that she was basically concentrating lead in her tea kettle as the water evaporated off. When the water content in a teapot lowers, most people simply add water to refill. Boiling turns that water to steam and it evaporates. Unfortunately, if the water contains even minimal amounts of lead (as was true in Connie's water supply), that lead does not evaporate. Instead it concentrates in the water. What's more, many commercial teas are also contaminated with lead, especially tea from highly polluted China, which produces about one-third of the tea consumed in the United States. Although in general, scientific research studies one chemical at a time, in reality, people are exposed to many different toxins simultaneously and sequentially. Without realizing it, Connie was absorbing a double dose of lead from the water and the tea.

Her condition was so severe that I asked her to move out of her home. Given the high concentrations of lead in Connie's water supply, it was absolutely crucial that she eliminate exposure to any possible source of lead whatsoever during her detox and recovery. Although the government has not yet defined sufficiently protective safety standards for absorption via inhalation (which occurs when showering) and skin contact (which occurs when bathing or washing dishes), these are two additional pathways through which toxins (like lead) can enter our bodies. During her recovery, I sought to make sure that Connie strictly avoid the lead-contaminated water, which could also be absorbed (albeit in minuscule amounts) through showering, washing, or wearing lead-contaminated clothing, as well as through cooking with, drinking from, or using utensils that could convey additional doses of lead into her system. I also immediately started her on an aggressive lead-detoxification program using the same strategies you will follow in the Toxin Solution.

Since she was otherwise healthy and led a healthy lifestyle, Connie responded quickly to treatment. Within about a week, her vision was back to normal. It took several more weeks for her energy to return completely. After her recovery, Connie began to look into a remediation plan for her home water supply to bring an end to any potential for reexposure.

With the right medical support, exposure to a single toxic substance (as in Connie's case) can be mitigated. But many people don't know what is afflicting them, and most conventional doctors don't either.

Exposure to lead is not as rare as most of us would like to believe. And as the American public learned recently, toxic exposures to substances like lead can occur even on a mass scale.

Mass Exposures

Consider the 2014 Flint, Michigan, disaster. The state government decided to save money by replacing Lake Huron as a water source.

Instead, they used water from a local river but did not address the problem of its being corrosive. Inevitably, the city's pipes corroded, causing lead to leach into Flint's drinking water. Houses built with leaded-copper water pipes added to the leaching of lead by the corrosive water. And when people drank that water, the lead entered their bodies. When public officials make cavalier decisions that fail to address public safety, people will suffer the ill effects. Along with other practitioners, I worked with public health officials to offer health support to the people of Flint. Millions of Americans are drinking water with lead levels above the public health limits.

Sadly, in most cases, communities do not find out about the toxins rampant in their area for years. The website Grist recently reported that "across the country, nine counties report that 10 percent or more of their population tested positive for lead poisoning, according to 2014 CDC data. Research by public health advocacy groups show that 11 New Jersey cities and two counties have higher lead levels than those in Flint, Michigan."[11] Nor does money earmarked to help always go to the afflicted families. Even though a percentage of paint sales in New Jersey was dedicated to helping families undertake lead remediation, the state's governor blocked the funding.[12]

You don't need to live in a house or community that has lead-contaminated pipes to be affected. Simply living under the flight paths of an airport can contaminate you, since lead is in 70 percent of U.S. airplane fuel, causing the release of over five hundred metric tons of lead a year.[13]

Although I use the example of lead, a supposedly banned substance, to illustrate the pervasiveness of exposures, the same is true of many other toxins. In helping me with the research for this book, a work colleague of mine discovered that a glass-making company just a few blocks from her home in Portland, Oregon, had been spewing arsenic and cadmium into its surroundings for forty years! The air quality across the street from the facility was found to be 49 times above the safe level for cadmium and 159 times above the safe level for arsenic. As you can see from figure 2.4, virtually the whole Portland area is deeply contaminated. This means more diabetes, lung cancer, osteoporosis, heart attacks—to name just a few of the diseases caused or aggravated by these toxic metals. You can bet there are a great many unrecognized areas of contamination like this one throughout the country, since widespread industrialization results in substantial local pollution.

Figure 2.4. **Arsenic and cadmium found in moss in Portland, Oregon**

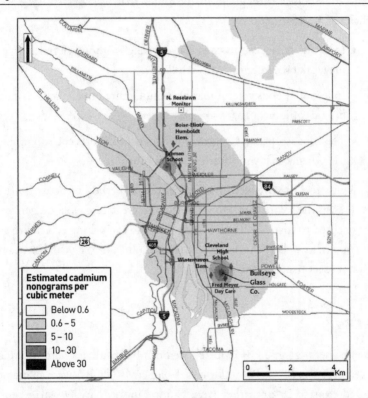

While there now exist better safeguards limiting toxin release, the damage has already been done. The key point here is that virtually everyone is being constantly exposed to toxins without being aware that this is happening. In Portland, although the people living in the immediate

---

Figure 2.4 source: www.opb.org/news/article/what-you-need-to-know-about-heavy-metals-pollution-in-portland.

area are the most exposed, simply driving through the city on Interstate 5 entails exposure to cadmium and arsenic. This is happening all over the country—Flint is not an isolated example.

Water supplies throughout the United States are contaminated not only with lead but also with arsenic, fluoride, industrial chemicals, carcinogens from fracking, and many other hazardous substances. Toxins enter our bodies through so many routes that we rarely think about them. A few examples:

- Inhalation: The transformer on your neighborhood electrical line may leak oil contaminated with PCBs.

- Ingestion: Foods you eat may be manufactured in facilities that use plastic equipment that leaks plasticizers.

- Topical absorption: Consumer products of all sorts contain toxic ingredients that you absorb through your skin.

As I stress many times, the most effective method of detoxification is to keep the toxins out. However, despite great care, you are going to be exposed to toxins and must consciously do everything you can to get them out, as well as encourage our elected officials to enact regulations that protect people from contamination.

PCBs

Some chemicals used in industry are both harmful and hard to avoid, even when banned. Polychlorinated biphenyls (PCBs) were manufactured from 1929 until they were banned in 1979. Why worry about chemicals banned thirty-eight years ago? Because food, lubricants, plastic containers, and carbonless copy paper manufactured before 1979 still contain them. Recently, the city of Portland, Oregon, sued the Monsanto Corporation for contaminating local bodies of water with PCBs, joining six other West Coast cities—Seattle, Spokane, Berkeley, Oakland, San Diego, and San Jose—in filing suit.

Ongoing Exposure

Even with the ban, nearly a half century later, PCBs continue to build up
in people's bodies. They are very hard to remove. Later on, I'll delve further into PCBs' health impacts, but for now, I'll just give a general picture: PCBs damage the immune, reproductive, nervous, and endocrine
systems. These man-made chemicals have been used in many buildings
and hundreds of industrial and commercial applications. Even if, as a
consumer, you have not intentionally purchased PCB-containing products, you might still be exposed to PCBs from:

- Paints, plastics, and rubber products
- Pigments, dyes, and carbonless copy paper
- Electrical equipment including voltage regulators, switches,
  reclosers, bushings, electromagnets, transformers, and capacitors
- Old appliances
- Oil used in motors and hydraulic systems
- Fluorescent light ballasts
- Cable insulation
- Thermal insulation material including fiberglass, felt, foam, and
  cork
- Adhesives and tapes
- Oil-based paint
- Caulking
- Plastics
- Floor finishes

Don't get me wrong: banning PCBs did benefit public health. The
ban helped to lower blood levels in the U.S. population. (See figure
2.5.) Nevertheless, products made before 1979 have been leaking
PCBs right up to today. The older a person is, the more PCBs he or

she has accumulated. (See figure 2.6.) Why? The body can quickly release some substances, but not others. PCBs are one class of chemicals that the body can't readily get rid of. So with each exposure you receive, you add to your existing PCB load. Over a lifetime, this load builds up.

Figure 2.5. **Banning PCBs resulted in the lowering of blood levels**

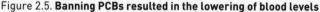

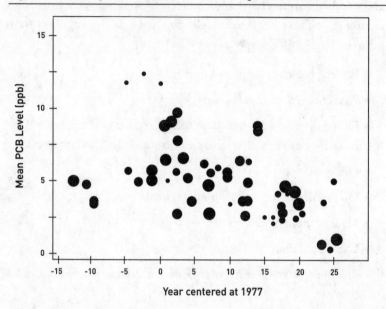

Year centered at 1977

I sometimes pessimistically wonder if the national average blood levels of these chemicals are decreasing mainly because older people, especially those with the highest levels, are simply dying off and so are no longer averaged with the rest of the population.

What Happens to the PCBs You Absorb?

PCBs inhibit the production of thyroid hormones, so people with elevated PCB levels feel fatigued all the time. But worse, PCB levels

Figure 2.5 source: N. B. Hopf, A. M. Ruder, and P. Succop, "Background levels of polychlorinated biphenyls in the U.S. population," *Science of the Total Environment* 407, no. 24 (2009): 6109–19.

Figure 2.6. **PCBs accumulate with age**

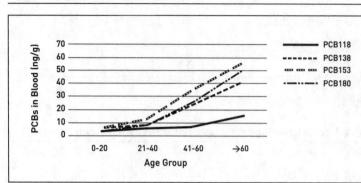

are now so high that they appear to cause a totally preventable 24 percent of all heart attacks![14] Yes, you've been told elevated cholesterol is the problem. But did your doctor tell you that cholesterol levels go up in proportion to the level of PCBs in your body? Cholesterol is normal, healthy, and required for health. PCBs are not. Rather, they and other toxins oxidize healthy cholesterol to unhealthy oxLDL (oxidized LDL) cholesterol, which is what actually damages arteries and causes heart attacks.

Fish are a common food source of PCBs. This is of real concern for women planning to have children. The more fish a woman eats (as measured by omega-3 fatty acids in her blood), the higher her level of PCBs. Unfortunately, a woman's PCB load doesn't stop with her. The good news is that breast-feeding lowers the mother's blood levels of PCB, OCPs, and other toxins. PCBs concentrate in breast milk, so nursing rids her body of these toxins. The bad news is that when her baby drinks that milk, the child takes in those toxins.

Why are fat-soluble toxins like PCBs so troubling for parents? Because they can:

Figure 2.6 source: B. Serdar, W. G. LeBlanc, J. M. Norris, and L. M. Dickinson, "Potential effects of polychlorinated biphenyls (PCBs) and selected organochlorine pesticides (OCPs) on immune cells and blood biochemistry measures: A cross-sectional assessment of the NHANES 2003–2004 data," *Environmental Health* 13 (2014): 114.

- Be excreted into a mother's breast milk.

- Be passed to the baby.

- Accumulate in the baby.

Perhaps one reason women who breast-feed have lower breast-cancer rates is that they are getting rid of these poisons.

Figure 2.7. **Breast-feeding decreases a woman's chemical toxin load**

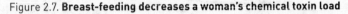

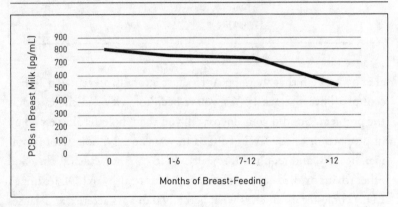

How Do PCBs Build over a Lifetime?

Without carefully looking at the scientific data, it is very hard for anyone to connect today's toxic exposure to long-range health effects. You might think, *Well, it's just one fish sandwich. How bad could that be?* Let's delve a bit deeper and look at some data. Over a period of *twenty-three years* (now there's a long-term study!), researchers measured the effects of PCBs.[15] (See figure 2.6.)

What did the researchers focus on in this study? Two things:

1. PCBs levels

2. Blood-sugar markers

Figure 2.7 source: H. Bjermo, P. O. Darnerud, S. Lignell, et al., "Fish intake and breastfeeding time are associated with serum concentrations of organochlorines in a Swedish population," *Environment International* 51 (2013): 88–96.

Blood-sugar markers indicate how well the insulin system is functioning. They provide a snapshot for where you are on the diabetes spectrum. (As I mentioned in chapter 1, research finds strong correlations between toxic load and blood-sugar dysregulation—that's not surprising, since many chemicals are insulin-receptor-site poisons.)

This study looked at young adults over a twenty-three-year period to determine the long-term impact of PCB exposure.[16] From the outset, the study included only participants who were *not* diabetic when it began. The researchers found that until the study participants reached the age of fifty, there were essentially no differences to be found between those with the lowest and highest PCB levels. In other words, the increasing toxin load appeared to have no discernible impact on younger people. But wait: the research also found that as the subjects aged past their mid-forties, their ability to adapt started rapidly decreasing with age. By age fifty, all the measures showed a very strong toxin-dose response: the higher the PCBs levels, the more impaired the blood-sugar regulation.

Figure 2.8. **Toxin effects with aging**

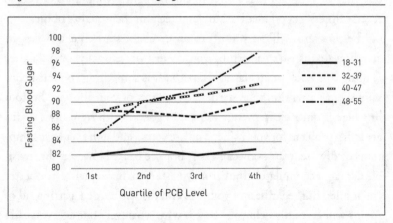

Figure 2.8 source: J. R. Suarez-Lopez, D. H. Lee, M. Porta, M. W. Steffes, and D. R. Jacobs Jr., "Persistent organic pollutants in young adults and changes in glucose related metabolism over a 23-year follow-up," *Environmental Research* 137 (February 2015): 485–94.

This finding reveals something that I believe applies to the overall understanding about toxic load and its impacts. Our wonderful bodies have a remarkable—but limited—ability to keep us healthy. After enough years of toxic overload, the body's adaptive capabilities eventually become too damaged. Basically, aging and its accompanying accumulated toxic load damage the DNA, resulting in progressively lower enzyme function. Over time, you lose your ability to adapt to this toxic environment.

The secret strength of naturopathic medicine, the medical philosophy I follow and teach, is twofold: our understanding of why people are sick and our knowledge of how to help them become healthy. The nine-week program I offer in the next chapters of this book will help you:

- Understand how toxic burden has become a primary cause of disease and ill health.

- Upgrade your detox capacity.

When I travel and lecture, I find that many physicians all over the world want to know more about detox. I've seen the scientifically validated detox program that I offer in this book help thousands of people reverse illness, get off medications, and reclaim their quality of life.

The program will get you off to an excellent start. But let's face it: avoiding toxins isn't something you do just occasionally, or only after reading this book or an alarming article. It is something you must consciously pay attention to every day for the rest of your life. The bottom line here is quite clear: even if you are in good health right now, toxins are still a problem for you. When you are young and don't yet have symptoms or disease, your body can easily bounce back. However, the invisible damage accumulates. The earlier you start toxin avoidance, the better the results. But regardless of your age and disease burden, getting rid of toxins will certainly help you. That is why, whatever your age, you can't wait another day to reduce your toxic load.

Toxic exposures drain your life energy, increase your risk of disease, and make you age more rapidly. You can't hold your breath to avoid inhaling the higher levels of mercury released by industrial activity. If you live in the Pacific Northwest, like me, you can get toxins from coal burning as far away as China.

In the next four chapters, you will access protocols to release the toxins you have absorbed. But beginning right now, and as you undertake the Nine-Week Toxin Solution, please limit your exposure.

Lessons from Four Generations

I am fortunate to be from a family that is relatively long-lived—one in which all my male ancestors that I am aware of outlived their wives (some had more than one wife!) by five to fifty years. In the photograph of my great-grandfather, grandfather, and father, the grumpy-looking kid at the end of the line is me. (See figure 2.9.) I had the chance to see what happens generation after generation as my forebears went from eating a healthy, nutrient-dense Mediterranean-type diet in a low-toxin environment to eating a poor-quality standard American diet, with no awareness of the importance of avoiding toxins. In fact, there was a growing load of toxin exposure from multiple sources, along with a progressive decrease in nutrient content of the foods we all were eating.

My great-grandfather lived to age ninety-five with no apparent health problems. He emigrated from the foothills of the Italian Alps in his forties and continued the diet and lifestyle he grew up with. He never saw a doctor in his life, walked briskly with no apparent pain or limitation, and would play strategy card games with me and never lose. This was quite frustrating for me, since as a precocious ten-year-old I would always beat all my friends playing strategy games. How could this old guy be beating me?! The answer is simple: his brain continued to work perfectly—no dementia, loss of short-term memory, or mental fogginess here.

After living alone independently for five years after his wife's death, he announced to the family that he was done with a great life, stopped eating, and was dead one week later. I don't know about you, but that is how

Figure 2.9. **The author with (from the left) his great-grandfather, grandfather, and father**

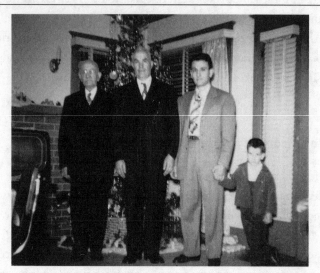

I want to go—fully functional until the very end, and then finishing life on my terms. As near as I can tell, he ate nutritious foods and had very little toxin exposure his whole life.

My grandfather was kind of halfway between my great-grandfather and father, having immigrated at age seventeen with my great-grandfather. He ate mostly, but not entirely, a Mediterranean-type diet, but with the poorer-quality foods grown in the United States (i.e., lower nutrient content and more toxins), he experienced, during the last twenty years of his life, the same growing toxic load all Americans are exposed to. He also lived to age ninety-five (and outlived two wives) but was in a nursing home his last ten years, with a modest amount of early chronic disease. Not debilitated, but not nearly as robust as his father.

And then there was my much-loved dad: Proud to "leave the old country behind," he ate the standard American diet, freely used the wonders of modern chemistry in his garage for maintaining the family house and property, and believed in prescription drugs for anything that ailed him. He also smoked for twenty years, but wisely decided this was bad for him and his family and simply quit cold-turkey one day. My dad developed dementia by age eighty-three and died at age eighty-eight, debilitated and suffering multiple serious chronic diseases. His living as long as he did was a testament to modern medicine and remarkable genetics. Heart disease, osteoporosis (requiring hip replacement), osteoarthritis, loss of short-term memory—the list of his health problems was long, as was the list of drugs his doctors prescribed for him. His problems didn't start suddenly when he "got old." By age sixty-five he already had significant osteoarthritis, osteoporosis, and heart disease. The first sign that his mental faculties were starting to deteriorate was that by his mid-sixties he could no longer drive safely at night.

As I write this, I am now older than that, and as seen in the photograph (figure 2.10), I tour all over the world on a motorcycle, with my wife on back. In many places, such as Australia, where this picture was taken, I have to drive on the left rather than on the right side of the road, where all my driving reflexes and experience developed.

Figure 2.10. **Author motorcycle-touring Australia in 2015**

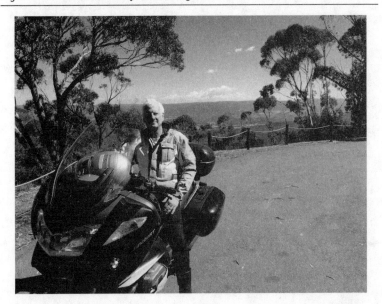

I became interested in nutrition when I graduated from college, and have eaten essentially organically since then. And while it is impossible to avoid all toxins anymore, I have led a relatively high-nutrition, low-toxin life since my early twenties.

Guess which of my forebears I am trying to emulate? Which of my forebears do you want to emulate? This is why this book is important to you and why you need to start my nine-week plan today. Maybe tomorrow. In any case, soon. Please, for the sake of your health and that of your children or children to be, don't delay.

3

The Two-Week Jumpstart Diet

Toxins are literally everywhere. And as you learned in chapter 2, only by understanding that there are both avoidable and hard-to-avoid toxins can you realistically limit your exposure. This chapter provides an overview of the toxic intrusion into our food. You'll also discover exactly how to steer clear of toxins in food and water through following the Two-Week Jumpstart Diet. Over the next two weeks on this diet, you will feel better immediately and will get the energy you need for the succeeding weeks of the Toxin Solution.

What will I do without my daily cheeseburger? some people wonder. Don't worry! The food plan I present in this chapter makes it easy to eat a nourishing, delicious, and contaminant-free diet that you will actually enjoy as you release toxins and regain health. And even though I want you to follow the entire program offered in this book, I'll let you in on a little secret: if you do nothing but follow the Two-Week Jumpstart Diet two to three times a year, you will experience a substantial improvement in your energy and well-being.

So, if you happen to pick up this book at a time when it's not convenient for you to do the full program, just follow this diet for two weeks.

Once you discover how easy it is, you will feel more confident, and motivated to make time in your schedule to do the complete program. But first, let's delve into why our once-healthy food supply is now an ugly conglomeration of poisons.

The Toxification of Food

Much of what people eat today can barely be classified as food. If you roam a supermarket, pick a few examples of food "products" right off the shelves, and take a good long look at what they contain, it will not surprise you that these highly processed products actually contain very little real food. Yes, they may look and even taste pretty good, despite their long list of mysterious ingredients. That's because they're dosed up with plenty of fat, salt, or sugar. Even if you avoid the central aisles and stick to the produce, dairy, and meat sections, you will still not have escaped from toxins in food. Why? Because bit by bit, a wide array of chemicals that human beings were never meant to consume has been introduced into the food supply. And sadly, even many once-nutritious foods are now made by industrialized agricultural entities that, while efficient, deliver a high load of toxins straight into our bodies.

Up until recently, the organic-farming movement had been making great headway in reversing the trend toward toxins in agriculture. But as the government weakens organic standards and subsidizes large corporations that farm thousands of acres with businesslike efficiency, it's becoming harder for everyone to find sources of healthy food. To make up for the depletion of our soil wrought by their megascale practices, agribusinesses pour a witch's brew of toxic chemicals onto fields—and into our nation's food supply. These substances include pesticides, contaminated synthetic fertilizers, and herbicides that contaminate not just the food they produce, but also the environment for miles and miles around.

Take apples, for example. Apples are as American as apple pie. But did you know that for the last several years, this quintessential American fruit has topped the "Dirty Dozen" list of the Environmental Working Group, a research and advocacy organization? The Dirty Dozen is a list of foods so contaminated that people must eat only the organic varieties. No longer "keeping the doctor away," apples contain more pesticides than any other fruit or vegetable. For starters, 80 percent of apples grown in the United States have a chemical called diphenylamine on them, which breaks down into cancer-causing nitrosamines. Growers spray apples with this chemical after the harvest to keep them from turning brown. Yes, the apples look great on the shelf, all red and shiny, but if you're smart, you'll leave them there!

"Nitrites and nitrates belong to a class of chemical compounds that have been found to be harmful to humans and animals," says researcher Dr. Suzanne de la Monte of Rhode Island Hospital. Increased levels of nitrates and nitrosamines are linked to increased incidence of Alzheimer's, Parkinson's, and type 2 diabetes. "We have become a nitrosamine generation," Dr. de la Monte says, adding that "more than 90 percent of these compounds that have been tested have been determined to be carcinogenic in various organs."[1]

No wonder the European Union banned American apples in 2012. So far, the U.S. apple industry has not responded to Europe's concerns. (In fact, if the new global trade deals like the Transatlantic Trade and Investment Partnership [TTIP] are passed, Europeans will soon *lose* their safer standards and healthier options.) Meanwhile, Americans sustain an ongoing toxic exposure through eating nearly ten pounds per person of raw apples every year. And even if the amount of diphenylamine in each apple is small, the risks mount with multiple servings of apples, apple juice, and applesauce in our own and our kids' diets. But the real problem is that this is not the only toxic chemical, and apples are not the only food that is contaminated. It all adds up.

Does that mean you can never again eat an apple? Certainly not. As you will see, they are included in the food plan you will find later in this chapter. But for certain foods—like apples—that are more contaminated with agricultural toxins, you must choose organic (or near-organic) varieties.

Will eating organic (or close to it) just for two weeks make a difference? Well, a family of five in Sweden did just that. As part of a study,
researchers put the family on a diet of conventionally grown food for one
week, followed by two weeks on organic foods. When researchers tested
the family members' urine for chemicals, they found that "concentrations of selected pesticides decreased by 95% when the family switched
to organic food."[2] The scientists' conclusion?

> Eating organic foods reduces the levels of a number of chemicals and sub-
> stances that we are exposed to through what we eat. This in turn reduces
> the risk of a long-term impact and combination effects. Choosing organic
> products also helps to reduce the spread of chemicals in the environment
> and protects those who work in the cultivation of fruit and vegetables.[3]

I've long recommended that my patients try this same experiment.
Switching to organic, even for two weeks, cures a variety of ills that people often fail to recognize as due to toxins. Researchers are now finding
a strong connection between the pesticides used to grow fruits, vegetables, and livestock feed, and virtually every dangerous illness. "Whatever
is happening is happening to everyone, suggesting an environmental
trigger," claims Robert H. Lustig, professor of clinical pediatrics at the
University of California, San Francisco.[4]

The good news is that blood levels of many toxins can decrease quickly.
The bad news is that it takes much, much longer to clear out the cell,
bone, and fat stores.

Sally's Story

Sally was a dedicated young mother with two beautiful little girls ages
four and six. Both Sally and her daughters were having problems with
energy—opposite problems. Sally reported feeling exhausted and "at
the end of her rope." Meanwhile, the little girls were bouncing off the
walls. At first glance, the girls' actions just seemed like youthful enthu-
siasm, but as I watched them noisily interact with other patients in

my waiting room, I began to suspect that they were right on the edge of hyperactivity.

Also suffering from insomnia and menstrual-cycle irregularities, Sally had seen her family MD several times, but he had nothing to recommend. As I watched her girls bounce around my office, irritating my patients, my first question was "How much sugar are you feeding them?"

Her answer: "None!" This surprised me. Sally did everything right for her family—avoiding junk food, giving a good multivitamin supplement, and offering a loving home environment. But where was she buying food? A recently published Seattle study measured the toxin levels in children. The study compared the toxic load of children who ate organic food from the Puget Consumers Co-op with that of those eating food from a regular grocery store. The neurotoxic pesticide levels of the children who ate conventionally grown foods were nine times higher![5]

Since Sally's physical exam was normal, rather than undertake expensive testing, Sally opted to start with the basics: properly grown healthy foods rich in nutrients and low in toxins. I recommended that she begin by shopping at the Puget Consumers Co-op. (I have been buying my food from this healthy food cooperative since 1970—back in the day when early organically grown foods did not look as nice as they do today thanks to a range of new growing techniques.)

When Sally objected that organic foods are more expensive, I asked her how that compared with the money she was spending to see doctors who weren't helping her. She got the message. A month later, she came back for a follow-up—and she was beaming. She had religiously followed my advice, and within just one week had noticed a difference. Not only was she feeling more energetic; she was also sleeping better. Her menstrual cycle had begun to normalize. Instead of hyperactively harassing my patients, her darling daughters were adorable, and calmer than on the previous visit, bringing smiles to my waiting patients. It really is often that simple; our bodies evolved to be healthy, if just given a chance.

Nowadays, accessing healthier food options is quite doable, thanks to both the food and informational resources we now have. If you can't go whole-hog and eat everything organic, you can concentrate your food purchases where they count most.

Easy Tools for Making Healthy Food Choices

One group that gets high marks in my book is the Environmental Working Group (EWG). Their online resources (at www.ewg.org) have helped millions of Americans face up to the realities of the toxins we consume and absorb. Let's take a look at their Dirty Dozen (plus two) food list. These are the foods with the heaviest doses of agricultural pesticides. If you want to unload your toxic burden and restore your health, you can concentrate your organic produce purchases on the following fruits and vegetables:*

1. Apples
2. Strawberries
3. Grapes
4. Celery
5. Peaches
6. Spinach
7. Sweet bell peppers
8. Nectarines (imported)
9. Cucumbers
10. Tomatoes
11. Snap peas (imported)
12. Potatoes
- Hot peppers
- Kale and collard greens

How Did Our Food Supply Get So Toxic?

About seventy years ago, the nature of the food we eat changed dramatically. The small family farms and backyard gardens that supplied our

---

* Kale, collard greens, and hot peppers do not meet traditional Dirty Dozen ranking criteria but were frequently found to be highly contaminated with organophosphate insecticides that are especially toxic to the human nervous system. The Environmental Working Group recommends that people who eat a lot of these foods buy organic instead.

food were superseded by industrial agriculture. Farmers stopped replenishing the soil, as they had been doing for thousands of years. Instead, they became dependent on synthetic fertilizers, which exhausted soil to maximize profits. Phosphates, a major ingredient in synthetic fertilizers, can release high levels of cadmium, a highly toxic metal, into the soil. Even worse, the fertilizers do not replace the trace minerals we need. The result is that the soil becomes progressively more depleted.

When we eat foods grown in mineral-depleted soil, they more easily absorb metals like cadmium. This metal is so toxic that the kidneys clear it as quickly as possible from the blood. Unfortunately, as we will discuss in chapter 6, it nevertheless gets stuck there, causing a lot of damage. In high concentrations, cadmium is even more toxic than lead or mercury and contributes to a large number of health conditions. Cadmium, for example, is linked to osteoporosis and even to the major killer diseases: heart disease, cancer, and diabetes. And, as you saw in table 1.3 in chapter 1, once cadmium gets into your body, it takes sixteen years to get rid of just half of it!

Another result of industrial agriculture was that farmers began to spray foods with insecticides on a large scale. Most of these insecticides, such as the organochlorines and organophosphates that I mentioned earlier, are neurological poisons.

Many foods are now inadvertently contaminated with herbicides. This happens because herbicides like glyphosate, used in genetically modified crops, are sprayed on the ground to keep down the growth of weeds. There are many ways these herbicides damage our bodies. For example, they disrupt the endocrine system by blocking both testosterone and estrogen receptor sites.[6] Even worse, they damage DNA, making cells age faster and become more susceptible to cancer.

Crops that have been genetically modified (GMOs) are designed to be resistant to the effects of specific herbicides. That is why farmers feel free to use them more and more in their fields. But while GMOs may perhaps be resistant to these poisons, humans and livestock are not!

While all of these so-called agricultural advances have increased commercial productivity, what winds up on your plate are foods depleted of nutrients, especially trace minerals. In place of the nutrients your body needs, you get toxic chemicals and metals. Poorer-quality, cheaper food may keep you alive, but it undermines health and actively induces disease.

Sheryl's Story

Sheryl was a college student struggling to maintain a C-plus grade average and dealing with low energy, weight gain, and acne. The last two had been lifelong problems. Sheryl regularly used both topical anti-acne lotions and potions and weight-loss products from the local pharmacy. She ate a poor diet of the cheapest food she could find, including—several times a week—a big box of frosted doughnuts from the grocery store. While the doughnuts were a cheap way to get calories, the energy boost she got from eating them was short-lived. The long-term effect of regular consumption of the doughnuts' food additives, chemical contaminants, sugars, and lack of nutrients was decreased energy, weight gain, and poor health.

Sheryl's problems were classic: nutritionally deficient foods contaminated with pesticides, aggravated by toxic health and beauty aids, unnecessary drugs, and a sedentary lifestyle. I advised her not to waste her very limited financial resources on expensive laboratory tests, so that she could instead spend her money on higher-quality food.

Sheryl decided that if she was going to spend her hard-earned money on my services, she was damn well going to do what I asked her to. I wish all my patients were so sensible! I warned her that her skin would get worse, possibly even for a couple of months, but I assured her that if she stuck with my program, her skin would ultimately get much better. My guidance for her was straightforward. I advised Sheryl to:

1. Stop putting toxic chemicals on her face and in her body.

2. Stop buying high-sugar, nutrient-depleted bakery products.

3. Spend her precious food budget on organic varieties of the foods she ate from the Dirty Dozen (plus two) list.

4. Inexpensively balance her diet and calories by buying the conventionally grown Clean 15 foods listed at www.ewg.org. (Obviously I'd have preferred for all her food to be organic, but she couldn't afford it.)

5. Find some exercise she liked. (It did not matter if it was simply walking or going to the free university gym a couple of times a week.)

Sheryl came back a month later, smiling. I could already see her starting to transform. Yes, her acne was worse, as I predicted, but within a week she had noticed her energy improving. After just one month, she was delighted to have lost five pounds. I congratulated her on her strong will and commitment to taking care of herself. Rather than spend her resources seeing me, I suggested she stay the course and not see me again for another three months, but I told her to feel free to give me a call at any time if she had any questions or needed any encouragement.

Over the next year her transformation was quite remarkable. Her skin totally cleared up, and she lost all of her extra twenty pounds. Her grades substantially improved, and she was accepted into a graduate master's degree program.

Although the solution for Sheryl was relatively simple, that does not mean it was always easy. When withdrawing from a drug that suppresses symptoms, the body overresponds before coming back to normal. The tough withdrawal from sugar, the embarrassing worsening of her acne, the feeling of uncertainty when her friends mocked her for "wasting money" on eating organically grown foods—it all took fortitude. But it was worth it. Because as her body reestablished proper function, the normal response was health.

As I mentioned in chapter 1, scientists and researchers now refer to pesticides and many other toxic chemicals as *diabetogens* and *obesogens*. Because of them, many foods once considered nutritious now lead to diabetes and obesity. Other research reveals that people with the highest levels of pesticide exposure (the top 10 percent) have a frighteningly twentyfold higher risk for diabetes. In fact, body load of pesticides is a better predictor of type 2 diabetes risk than any other factor. These chemicals go directly into the body's insulin-receptor sites and block them. As a result, insulin—the key hormone that regulates and normalizes blood sugar—can no longer perform its crucial job.

Pesticide toxins also stimulate enzymes that convert calories into fat—and your body's fat is precisely where toxins are stored. This means that when you start losing weight, your fat cells release higher concentrations of toxins, making both weight loss and detoxification more difficult and uncomfortable. That is why it's essential that detox be approached with caution and care, through the plan I offer in this book. As noted earlier, the goal is to get the toxins out quickly, but also safely.

Weight gain, obesity, prediabetes, and diabetes aren't the only aftermaths of toxic exposure. As I mentioned in chapter 1, Americans have lost a total of 41 million IQ points due to exposure to lead, mercury, and organophosphate (OP). OPs act as a poison to the nervous systems of insects, plants, and humans. It's a tragedy that we've gotten to the point where our foods are poisoning us rather than simply nourishing us as they should.

Supplanting crucial nutrients and exchanging them for toxic metals and chemicals is not a good trade if you seek health. If you follow no other feature of the Toxin Solution, I hope you will undertake this plan. It's core to restoring and maintaining your health.

The Two-Week Jumpstart Diet

Your detoxification capability—your ability to detox effectively and safely—depends on what you eat. The nutrients that your body uses to rid yourself of your built-up toxic load are often deficient for all the reasons I've mentioned. Fortunately, you can change that. For example, fiber is critical to the detoxification process, because it binds toxins in the gut and helps to carry them out of the body. In the past, humans ate about 100 to 150 grams of fiber every day. Currently, people in Western countries eat about 15 grams of fiber every day; and that figure is even less—12 grams per day—among non-Hispanic blacks.[7] Without enough fiber, the toxins are reabsorbed. That's why on my plan you will consume more fiber. And that's just the beginning.

Frankly, I am going to ask a lot of you over the next two weeks. For some, the first week may seem a little difficult. As you withdraw from the toxins to which you are habituated, you might notice some changes. Your breath might smell worse. Your energy might dip. You might feel cranky. Your friends might deride you for making yourself uncomfortable for no apparent reason. However, I guarantee that by the second week you will clearly feel better and will start to realize just how much healthier you can be.

According to my dear friend the brilliant clinician Sid Baker, MD, functional and naturopathic medicine focus on getting into your body what you uniquely need, and getting out of your body what you uniquely don't need. The Two-Week Jumpstart Diet will help you to do both.

The Don'ts

As I mentioned in chapter 2, people commonly welcome toxins into their bodies because they don't recognize that they are there.

On my plan you will stop consuming the following:

- Processed foods
- Gluten-containing foods
- Dairy products
- Beef and chicken
- Farmed fish
- The "Dirty Dozen" produce items
- Soy products

- Refined foods and sweeteners

- Alcohol and recreational drugs

- Salt

- Water that has not been purified or proven to be clean

Let's take a deeper look at why, in order to relieve your toxic burden and restore your health, it's essential to eliminate these "don'ts."

Processed Foods

Most so-called foods on the supermarket shelves contain harmful chemicals and additives, usually to make them look and taste better or last longer. But it's a bargain with the devil. Potassium bromate added to bread to increase its volume is carcinogenic, as is the butane added to chicken nuggets to keep them "fresh." BHA and BHT extend the shelf life of foods while probably shortening ours: both are linked to cancerous tumor growth. Sodium benzoate added to carbonated drinks may damage your DNA. And chemicals are being added not just to processed foods but to meat, dairy products, and even produce. The sodium nitrate added to processed meat (like sliced turkey and salami) to stop bacterial growth is linked to cancer in humans.

That's not all. Tartrazine dye is added to cheese to make it yellow, since cows are no longer eating grass high in colorful carotenoids. Unfortunately, tartrazine increases the risk of diseases such as asthma. Other chemicals help foods keep their color—like the sulfites added to dried fruit to keep it from turning brown. Those unable to effectively detoxify these sulfites (like me) experience allergies and nasal congestion, and they cause about 10 percent of asthma. And because these food products are often so devoid of nutrition and tastiness, food scientists devise flavoring agents to fool your taste buds.

Monosodium glutamate supposedly enhances flavor (it must be an acquired taste!), but unfortunately, it also enhances the risk of nerve and heart damage and seizures. And take note: while you may have sworn off MSG in your Chinese food, this shady character has a dozen aliases. Glutamic acid, hydrolyzed protein, autolyzed protein, autolyzed yeast extract, textured protein, and maltodextrin are just a few of them. The flavorings industry itself has estimated that over a thousand flavoring ingredients have the potential to act as respiratory hazards to the workers who are handling them, due to their volatility and irritant properties.

This survey of additives (for a complete list, see chapter 8, page 205) would not be complete without those artificial sweeteners luring us with their promise that we can enjoy dessert without the calories. Aspartame and saccharin have both been linked to cancer. Splenda, the best-selling sweetener on the market, has the added virtue of remaining stable when heated, which makes it "good" for baking. But though Splenda may make a very nice muffin, when heated it releases chloropropanols—a form of dioxin. According to the World Health Organization, dioxin, a key component in Agent Orange, "can cause reproductive and developmental problems and damage the immune system, interfere with hormones, and also cause cancer."[8]

Gluten-Containing Foods

Wheat may be "the staff of life," but it's not a good food choice for most people. The main protein in many grains, such as wheat, rye, and barley, is gluten. It's what gives bread and other foods that elastic, chewy texture and great smell when baking. But while gluten is good for bread, many find it's not good for the lining of their intestines. In susceptible people, gluten can inflame the gut and make it too permeable, which allows toxins into the bloodstream. And an extreme form of gluten intolerance known as celiac disease can lead to malnutrition and weight loss. One in every 141 people in the United States is diagnosed with celiac disease. (If you include undiagnosed cases, the number is probably twice as high.) Even without celiac disease, many people experience reactions to wheat. The most obvious food allergies are those of the immediate hypersensitivity type. When you eat this type of allergic food, you get symptoms, well, immediately. Experiencing hives, an asthma attack, a runny nose, or even fatigue after eating a food makes the connection obvious. These allergies can be confirmed with skin testing or allergen-specific immunoglobulin E (IgE) blood tests. Far more difficult to recognize are delayed reactions to specific foods. Since such reactions can take hours or even days to manifest, they are difficult to recognize. Standard skin tests typically don't measure them.

Whether or not you are allergic, it pays to avoid wheat when you are trying to restore your organs and your detox capacity. That's why you can start by avoiding gluten-containing products on the Two-Week Jumpstart Diet. Begin by carefully reading labels; you won't always see gluten listed, but you will see words like *flour, triticale, triticum, semolina, durum, Kamut, wheat, rye,* and *barley* that should tip you off. The problems some people have with grains are worsened when farmers breed wheat to increase its gluten content, or use antibiotics, which disrupt gut flora.

From the clinical point of view, by avoiding wheat, rye, and barley, over 75 percent of my patients who were suffering from chronic diseases improved dramatically; some were even totally cured. (Those with the most severe reactions also had to avoid corn, rice, and oats.) I can recount hundreds of stories of people who received little or no benefit from years of conventional treatment but were totally cured of rheumatoid arthritis, asthma, eczema, chronic vaginitis, inflammatory bowel disease, and chronic ear infections (in children)—simply by cutting out grains.

A Mysterious Depression

Ed was a therapist I often referred patients to. One reason he was so good at his job was his own personal history of depression. Therapy and medication hadn't helped him overcome this, so Ed consulted me to see if I could find a nutritional reason for his problem. He had a relatively good diet, took an excellent multivitamin and mineral supplement, and had no apparent physical problems. I was mystified, but since I had seen many patients get better through the simple act of giving up wheat, I told him to avoid wheat and all other grains for four days. Following my instructions, on the morning of the fifth day, he ate one piece of bread—with stunning results. A half hour after eating the bread, Ed described feeling "high" and became hyperactive. After two hours of this, he became so depressed he couldn't get out of bed for the rest of the day. This extreme reaction was such a surprise to him that he repeated the challenge test a week later, with the same, though less intense, results. As you might expect, Ed religiously avoided wheat from then on. His bouts of depression totally disappeared.

Most people find they are able to eat gluten-containing foods again after completing the two-week plan. However, based on genetics, 20 percent of people should *never* eat wheat, and 60 percent should not eat it more than a few times a week. For that lucky 20 percent, wheat causes no problems, and they get the benefit of the important nutrients and fiber in whole grains. In appendix G, you will find resources and information for testing to find out which category you are in.

Dairy Products

Mother's milk is a natural food for infants, but once we leave infancy most people's intestinal cells stop producing lactase, the enzyme needed to digest milk sugar. Some people continue to produce lactase into adulthood but lose it later in life. Lactose intolerance is especially common in adults of African, Mexican, or Mediterranean descent. Sometimes it can be difficult to recognize, because people don't expect foods they normally eat to suddenly become a problem.

Maria's Story

Episodes of indigestion brought Maria, a forty-five-year-old Hispanic mother of three, to my office. The discomfort came a few hours after meals and gradually disappeared. In the previous few months her symptoms

had become more frequent and longer-lasting. I suspected lactose intolerance. Maria doubted that this was the problem, since she had been eating dairy products her whole life without apparent trouble. When her
symptoms disappeared after four days of scrupulously avoiding all dairy
products, she was pleasantly surprised, but not totally convinced. Just to
be sure, a week later she drank a glass of milk—and suffered the worst
symptoms she'd ever had!

Maria's was an extreme case. Eliminating all dairy foods, such as milk,
cream, butter, yogurt, cheese, and ice cream, does not have to be a permanent feature of your diet; it's just for these two weeks, when it will unbur-
den your liver and help your gut heal. And unless you eat organic dairy
products, you are also giving your system a two-week break from the hormones and antibiotics that are fed to milk-producing livestock. Cows are
fed large amounts of these drugs, usually through a slow-release pellet in
their ears, to stimulate milk production and ward off infection. Some of
these pellets also contain insecticides to keep flies away.[9] Livestock also
eat grains raised with pesticides and herbicides. All of this gets passed
on to you with the cheddar slices and Greek yogurt and cottage cheese.

On the two-week plan, you will just say no to dairy products.

Beef and Chicken

Staying away from beef and chicken for two weeks is another short-term
measure. Cows raised for slaughter also get ear pellets that deliver andro-
gens, estrogens, and progesterones to enhance growth. The pellets, along
with the ears, are discarded when the cow is slaughtered.[10] The corn fed
to cattle to make them bigger, and their meat more deliciously fatty, also
makes their meat high in omega-6 fatty acid arachidonic acid, which promotes inflammation. To counter this, you need more anti-inflammatory
omega-3 fatty acids. Fish is a good source of this commonly deficient
fatty acid.

Many people consider chicken a healthy food. I consider it to be a
good protein source. However, conventionally raised chickens have elevated levels of arsenic due to the drugs and chemicals used in their production.[11] In fact, the CDC has listed arsenic as the worst toxin in the

United States, largely because of its presence in chicken. Chicken may also be contaminated with salmonella.

In contrast, eggs from free-range chickens are an excellent source of protein, and, when combined with organically grown vegetables, provide a much healthier option.

Farmed Fish

Don't be fooled by claims that "all fish is good for you." Large fish (like tuna and swordfish) are virtually always contaminated with high levels of mercury. Many fish are also contaminated with PCBs. Even though food companies market farm-raised fish under harmless-sounding names like "Atlantic salmon," these fish are fed food contaminated with persistent organic pollutants (POPs). It's not surprising they generally have high toxin levels as can be seen in figure 3.1.[12] Along with salmon, tilapia, rainbow trout, and striped bass are often farm raised. Read the label—and choose "wild-caught" instead. More expensive but much healthier. And, you will soon notice how much better wild fish taste.

The fish oils made from farmed fish are also highly contaminated. I am a great believer in taking fish oils for health, but make sure they come from reputable sources!

Note that farmed fish have more total fat than wild fish. And stored in the fat of those supposedly healthy fish exists a shocking assortment of toxins, including DDT. Yes, DDT. Even though it was banned in 1972, it persists in the environment, and makes its way into farmed fish. It's especially scary that some farmed salmon also have a stunning 7,200 ng (nanograms) of PCBs per serving! Farmed fish may have less mercury, but the benefit is far outweighed by very high levels of these other chemical toxins.

Remember, these chemicals are extremely difficult to get out of the body, with half-lives ranging from months to years. One serving or even ten servings is not a problem. But eating farm-raised fish even once a week (the least amount you need to eat to get enough omega-3 fatty acids) results in a huge toxic load.

In contrast, wild-caught fish have low levels of toxins. But large fish, even wild-caught, eat other smaller fish in the wild, and tend to bioaccumulate mercury that way. The best fish are wild-caught sardines and salmon, which are high in omega-3 fatty acids and low in mercury.

Figure 3.1. **Median concentrations of HCB, HCHs, DDTs, PBDEs, and marker PCBs per gram of fat in salmon, feed, and fish oil samples**

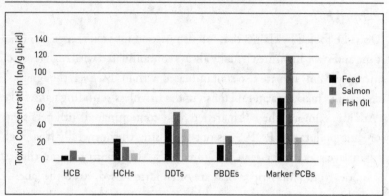

The sad reality is that PCBs and mercury aren't the only chemicals polluting fish. Recent testing found a "medicine chest of common drugs" in juvenile salmon—and in the waters of Puget Sound, Washington. A local news report noted that "most of the chemicals detected aren't monitored or regulated in wastewater, and there is little or no established science on the environmental toxicity of the vast majority of the compounds detected."[13] These included the following:

- Flonase
- Aleve
- Tylenol
- Paxil

- Valium
- Zoloft
- Tagamet
- OxyContin

- Darvon, Cipro, and other antibiotics

Even if you haven't been prescribed these medications, even if you conscientiously avoid antibiotics, you could be imbibing them anyway.

Figure 3.1 source: M. N. Jacobs, A. Covaci, and P. Schepens, "Investigation of selected persistent organic pollutants in farmed Atlantic salmon (*Salmo salar*), salmon aquaculture feed, and fish oil components of the feed," *Environmental Science & Technology* 36 no. 13 (2002): 2797–805.

Table 3.1. **Mercury Levels in Seafood**

	SPECIES	MEAN (PPM)	RANGE (PPM)
Large fish with high levels of methyl mercury	Tilefish (also called golden or white snapper)	1.45	0.65–3.73
	Swordfish	1.00	0.10–3.22
	King mackerel	0.73	0.30–1.67
	Shark	0.96	0.05–4.54
Fish or shellfish that may at times contain high levels of mercury	Grouper (Mycteroperca)	0.43	0.05–1.35
	Tuna (fresh or frozen)	0.32	ND–1.30
	Lobster, northern (American)	0.31	0.05–1.31
	Red snapper*	0.60	0.07–1.46
	Trout, freshwater*	0.42	1.22 (max.)
	Trout, seawater*	0.27	ND–1.19
Fish or shellfish with much lower levels of mercury	Halibut	0.23	0.02–0.63
	Sablefish	0.22	ND–0.70
	Pollock	0.20	ND–0.78
	Tuna (canned)	0.17	ND–0.75
	Crab, blue	0.17	0.02–0.50
	Crab, Dungeness	0.18	0.02–0.48
	Crab, tanner	0.15	ND–0.38
	Crab, king	0.09	0.02–0.24
	Scallops	0.05	ND–0.22
	Catfish	0.07	ND–0.31
	Salmon (fresh, frozen, or canned)	ND	ND–0.18
	Oysters	ND	ND–0.25
	Shrimp	ND	ND

PPM = parts per million
ND = not detectable
*Based on limited sample sizes; therefore, these figures have a much greater degree of uncertainty

Table 3.1 source: Data from U.S. Food and Drug Administration, Center for Food Safety and Applied Nutrition, "Mercury Levels in Seafood Species," May 2001.

Healthiest Fruits and Vegetables

Earlier in this chapter you read about the Dirty Dozen produce types (page 74). In terms of pesticide levels, the worst fruits on that list are clearly apples, strawberries, and grapes, so be sure to eat these organically. The menu plans in this chapter all call for organically grown varieties of these fruits.

The worst vegetables on the Dirty Dozen list are celery, spinach, and kale. This is especially frustrating, since spinach and kale are among the most nutrient-dense foods you can eat. Kale not only has the highest nutrient-to-calorie ratio of virtually any food; it also has critical phytonutrients that promote detoxification in the liver. Unfortunately, nonorganic kale also has the highest levels of organophosphate pesticides, which are extremely neurotoxic. As mentioned earlier (page 78), high levels of these toxins are associated with decreased IQ. They are also associated with increased ADHD in children. As you can see in figure 3.2, adults in the 76–90 percent levels of organochloride pesticides show a risk of dementia 2.5 times higher than that of those with the lowest levels. Those in the top 5 percent level of exposure have a whopping 6.5-fold increase in risk for dementia.

Figure 3.2. **Associations between organochlorine pesticides and cognition in U.S. elders, 1992–2002**

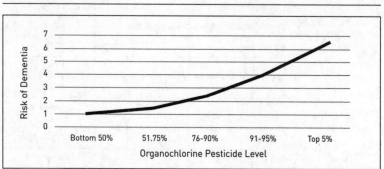

Figure 3.2 source: K. S. Kim, Y. M. Lee, H. W. Lee, D. R. Jacobs Jr., and D. H. Lee, "Associations between organochlorine pesticides and cognition in U.S. elders: National Health and Nutrition Examination Survey 1999–2002," *Environment International* 75 (2015): 87–92.

Nutrient Deficiency

Our bodies are basically enzyme machines. We use these special proteins to:

- Digest our food.
- Convert protein, carbohydrates, and fats into energy.
- Produce our hormones.
- Make reproduction possible.
- Create the messages that make our brains work.

In order to perform these and countless other functions, we need ample enzymes—and enzymes are made using key nutrients from the foods we eat. What does it take to make an enzyme? Enzymes have two components: an inactive protein skeleton, and a "cofactor" that activates it. Almost all the enzyme cofactors are vitamins or minerals. If you don't get generous quantities of vitamins and minerals from food, your enzymes won't work, or will work inadequately. That undermines health and leaves the body more susceptible to toxins. But most of the food

Figure 3.3. **Loss of minerals in food the past fifty years**

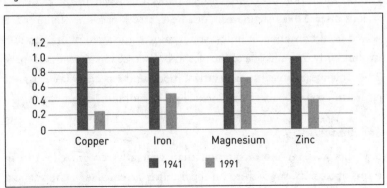

Figure 3.3 source: D. Thomas, "A study on the mineral depletion of the foods available to US as a nation over the period 1940 to 1991," *Nutrition and Health* 17, no. 2 (2003): 85–115.

grown today by huge agribusinesses is not providing the critical trace minerals and vitamins our enzymes need.

As you can see in figure 3.3, the amount of copper in food, for example, was almost 80 percent lower in 1991 than it was fifty years earlier! I suspect that if we had data from over the past one hundred years, the numbers would show an even greater disparity.

Cadmium

But it's even more serious than that. Forty years ago, I read a study that gave me an important insight. When plants are grown in nutrient-depleted soils, they actually absorb toxic metals *more easily*. The study looked at spinach grown on zinc-depleted soil. The results were clear: low zinc in the soil resulted not only in less zinc in the spinach but, even worse, more cadmium. That's because cadmium replaces zinc in critical enzymes when zinc levels are low. And once the cadmium levels get high enough, these enzymes will be poisoned. That exchange of unhealthy cadmium for healthy zinc is taking place right now in food crops across this country. Exactly the same thing is happening in our body.

Cadmium is one of those sneaky toxins that produce almost no symptoms (unless you sustain a high level of industrial exposure). The first clinical indication of its presence at dangerous levels in the body is a serious disease like osteoporosis, or a heart attack or kidney failure. You would not know about it unless you measured the amount of cadmium in your body through one of the methods discussed in appendix B (page 229). If you eat conventionally grown foods, and especially if you smoke cigarettes, you probably carry a toxic load of cadmium in your body.

Soy Products

Soy allergy is far more common than generally recognized. And in terms of toxicity, soy is third on the list after arsenic-laden chicken and farmed fish.

While soybeans have a number of nutritional benefits, they absorb a lot of cadmium when grown with high-phosphate fertilizers. A Seattle study found that soy products now have so much cadmium that their consumption causes an incredible 20 percent of the osteoporosis in women.[14] And when you think soy, it's not just tofu and soy sauce. Today we have the following soy products:

- Soy milk
- Soy protein powder
- Soy cheese
- Soy ice cream
- Soy pasta
- Soy burgers
- Soy protein bars
- Soy pizza

Most people are unlikely to consume more than one serving a day of broccoli. But soy food, because of its neutral taste, has become a staple.[15] Soy is also widely used in the feed for cattle, chickens, and pigs, serving as a secondary source for those who eat meat and dairy. Even if you aren't actively eating tofu and other soy products, soy oil is hard to avoid. It's present in countless processed foods, from mayo to chips to pudding. That's another good reason to avoid processed foods—as well as much meat and all dairy.

There is another big concern about soy in the food supply. Ninety-nine percent of the soy Americans consume is GMO. (Unlike sixty-four other countries, the United States does not require labeling of GM foods.) Why is this of concern?

There have been sharp increases in the amounts and numbers of chemical herbicides applied to GM crops. And further increases—the largest in a generation—are scheduled to occur in the next few years. GMOs were genetically modified to allow them to resist herbicides, so larger amounts of them can be sprayed on GMO crops to kill weeds. Unfortunately, those herbicides affect not only weeds; they damage us as well. According to the *New England Journal of Medicine,* "the International Agency for Research on Cancer (IARC) has classified glyphosate, the herbicide most widely used on GM crops, as a 'probable human carcinogen' and has classified a second herbicide, 2,4-dichlorophenoxyacetic acid (2,4-D), as a 'possible human carcinogen.'"[16]

There is a lot of controversy about whether GMOs are good for us or not. But there is no dispute that they lead to much higher levels of chemical contamination. A research team in France has shown that although glyphosate-containing herbicides like Roundup are touted as safe, that finding overlooks the real problem: their inactive—and much more toxic—constituents aren't disclosed.[17] In fact, this research team found that when you consider those ingredients, Roundup is one thousand times more toxic than pure glyphosate.[18] No wonder the European Union is considering dramatically restricting its use. Come on, U.S. government, what about you? You are supposed to be protecting us, not the big chemical companies!

Refined Foods and Sweeteners

Certain "foods" have their nutrient content and fiber stripped away to make them more attractive or tastier or more easily digestible. Flour, stripped of its germ and fiber and then ground into a very fine powder, is a common example. Another refined food, table sugar, has been linked to the following health issues:

- Obesity
- Diabetes
- Cardiovascular disease
- Dementia
- Macular degeneration
- Tooth decay

Even natural foods that have a high sugar content, like fruits, fruit juice, and honey, can cause blood sugar to fluctuate wildly when consumed to excess.

Sugar is remarkably addictive. For most of humankind throughout all of human history, getting sufficient calories was critical for survival. This is still true in many parts of the world, though it's quite the opposite in the United States today. A special biochemical pathway in the brain rewards us for eating sugar by releasing dopamine,[19] the very same molecule activated in heroin and cocaine use (and leading to addiction) in all populations studied.[20] If you don't believe that sugar is truly addictive, try to stop eating all forms of refined sugar for two days and watch what you crave. Toxins come in many forms, and even normal molecules, when taken in at high dosages, can cause problems.

Now, having said all that, I am *not* suggesting using synthetic sugar substitutes, like Splenda, saccharin, aspartame, and high-fructose corn syrup. They are all foreign chemicals your body must detoxify.

I consider high-fructose corn syrup (HFCS), widely used in sodas and fruit-flavored drinks, to be a toxin. HFCS, which is cheaper than sugar cane because of government corn subsidies, carries an even worse risk than sugar, including a link to fatty liver disease, obesity, and diabetes. I'll discuss this issue further in the next chapter.

Small amounts of sugar are not a problem. But when the average person gets 20 percent of his or her daily calories from sugar, that excess consumption is a problem. I suggest you get no more than 5 percent of your calories from sugar. (A teaspoon of sugar contains 16 calories. So a typical woman should not eat more than 10 teaspoons of sugar, a typical man not more than 15 teaspoons. Yes, that seems like a lot, but the average person consumes 25 to 50 teaspoons of sugar a day!)

Noreen's Story

Noreen had developed obesity and type 2 diabetes; her pancreas wore out from having to produce excessive insulin. To assess what was going on, I ordered certain tests that measure blood sugar every five minutes over a twenty-four-hour period. Figure 3.4 shows her blood sugar while eating a typical poor-quality diet, low in fiber and high in sugar. Every time Noreen ate a food with refined sugar, her blood sugar soared, only to then drop quickly, making her voraciously hungry.

Over a period of a few months, Noreen cleaned up her diet, ate more fiber-rich foods like beans and lentils, and started taking 6 grams of fiber (PGX) two to three times a day. The difference was dramatic.

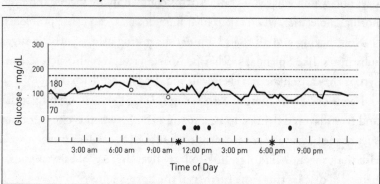

Figure 3.4. **Blood sugar levels for Noreen, a type 2 diabetic, taken every five minutes for a twenty-four-hour period**

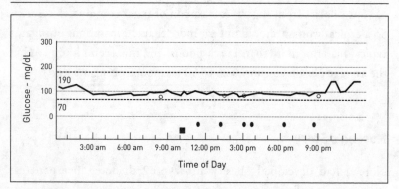

Figure 3.5. **Blood sugar levels for Noreen six months after her diabetes disappeared**

After six months of detoxification, Noreen lost thirty pounds *and no longer had diabetes!* Not only did the fiber stabilize Noreen's blood sugar; it also helped her get rid of the toxins, which had poisoned her insulin-receptor sites. Diabetes is a diagnosis, a label. By understanding disturbed insulin functions, Noreen was able to avoid the foods and the toxins that produced and worsened this condition.

Figure 3.4 and figure 3.5 source: Michael R. Lyon, MD, ABOM, Medical Director, Medical Weight Management Center, Coquitlam, British Columbia.

Almost 50 percent of the population has diabetes or prediabetes—both of which are almost entirely due to poor diet, lack of exercise, and toxins. Avoiding refined sugar can help ensure that your blood-sugar level remains steady throughout the day—neither too high nor too low nor changing rapidly.

Alcohol and Recreational Drugs

Along with the toxins in your food that you will be eliminating on the Two-Week Jumpstart Diet, I also suggest that you eliminate alcohol to excess, marijuana to excess, and any drugs that aren't necessary to keep you alive. (But check with your doctor before eliminating or reducing the dosage of any prescription drug.)

It's well known that alcohol, in moderation, provides some protection from heart disease. But alcohol is a toxin. That's the bottom line. The reason alcohol is used to preserve dead specimens is that it kills microorganisms. To detoxify alcohol, your liver uses up an essential antioxidant called glutathione. (Glutathione is the key molecule your body uses to get rid of most chemical toxins.) In excessive amounts, alcohol will damage your body, in addition to impairing your judgment and making your thinking fuzzy and your movements less coordinated. Chronic excessive drinking can also cause the following issues:

- High blood pressure
- Stroke
- Irregular heartbeat
- Degeneration of the heart muscle
- Weakening of the pancreas
- Weakening of the immune system
- Lowered resistance to infection
- Increased chance of getting cancer of the liver, mouth, esophagus, throat, or breast

In later weeks of the program, I will explore in detail how alcohol weakens the organs of detoxification. For now, here is a good rule of thumb: women should drink a daily maximum of one to two ounces of alcohol; for men, the maximum is two to three ounces.

Salt

Excess salt acts as a toxin in the body. When you eat too much salt, you impair your body's ability to produce glutathione. The higher your salt intake, the less your kidneys are able to detoxify because they are wasting their capacity getting rid of the excess sodium and chloride. More important, researchers now think that lifelong consumption of salt at the current typical amount of 3.4 grams per day may be the key reason people's kidneys degenerate as they age. The salt seriously stresses the kidneys to work overtime to get rid of the excess. This progressive loss of kidney function not only makes excretion of toxins more difficult; it's also a key factor in premature aging. So on my plan you will also eliminate salt. After two weeks, you will be surprised at how good your food tastes without it—but during the first few days you will most certainly notice its absence.

Unpurified Water

Unfortunately, at least 10 percent of U.S. public water supplies are contaminated with arsenic. In areas that burn coal for energy, the water also contains undesirable toxins like mercury. Water supplies near large, conventional farms contain pesticides and herbicides. Unless your water has been tested and found to be pure, I recommend that you err on the side of caution by drinking only tested and purified water. You can ensure that your water is safe in several ways:

1. If your water comes from a well, connect with Doctors Data (www.doctorsdata.com), which will test your water for toxic metals. Great Plains Laboratory (www.greatplainslaboratory .com) will test for chemicals.

2. If you drink municipal water, ask your city to provide an analysis. Be sure they are actually testing for metals, not just reporting total mineral content, which typically looks only at calcium and magnesium.

3. If you live in a house and want to be very careful, install a whole-house carbon block filter. This filters out all chemical toxins (except probably fluoride) from the water you drink and use for bathing. It's expensive, but fortunately, it's a one-time expense.

You can find information about getting your water tested or treated in appendix G.

The Do's

In this chapter so far, I have covered how to limit toxic exposure by avoiding certain foods and substances. But it's also necessary to focus on what you *should* eat. I do not want you to be fasting. I want you to be super clean in your eating and provide your body with the kind of nourishment that will help it detox naturally. To accomplish this, you should:

- Drink at least four quarts of clean water every day.
- Take a high-quality multistrain probiotic.
- Take a high-quality multivitamin and mineral supplement.
- Include more fiber in your diet.
- Eat half a pound of brassica-family foods every day.
- Eat lots of vegetables from the "Clean 15."
- Eat real, unprocessed food.
- Use turmeric but not pepper.
- Use oils carefully.

Drink at Least Four Quarts of Clean Water Every Day

Our kidneys play a major role in detoxification. They do this by removing water-soluble toxins from the body to be excreted via the urine. In the detox process, which I discuss in chapters 5 and 6, these toxins are bound to specific molecules (like glutathione, in the case of chemical toxins, and n-acetyl cysteine, in the case of methyl mercury from fish). Water is key to this process, because it helps to dilute the toxins, lowering their concentration in the urine so that they are less toxic to the kidneys. That is why you will be drinking four quarts of water daily.

Take a High-Quality Multistrain Probiotic

Choose a good probiotic, one that contains both *Lactobacillus* and *Bifidobacterium* strains. (Taking this supplement may give you more gas for a few days—a harmless side effect as your body adapts to reestablishing a healthy flora.)

Include More Fiber

The first day, take 1 gram of fiber three times a day. Increase to 2 grams the second day. The rest of the first week, take 3 grams of dietary fiber three times a day. Be sure to consume a full glass of water (this is included in your four-quart calculation) each time you take the fiber supplement. The second week, increase to 6 grams three times a day, again with plenty of water. And, of course, eat more foods rich in fiber, like beans and lentils.

Increase Brassicas and Healthy Vegetables

Eat half a pound of brassica-family foods every day (any color cabbage, broccoli, Brussels sprouts, cauliflower, and kale.) *These vegetables must be organically grown.* It's okay to cook them, but they must first be chopped up so the enzymes needed to produce the healthy, anticarcinogenic compounds that facilitate liver detox can be activated. (After chopping, wait at least five minutes before cooking, because heat will kill the enzymes. The compounds themselves are heat stable, so once they are produced, the enzymes are no longer needed.)

> ### Fiber
> There are quite a number of healthy fibers. I especially like flaxseed powder, pectin, alginate, and a combination fiber called PGX. (Full disclosure: I consult for Natural Factors, the manufacturer of PGX.) I recommend fiber supplements because it is much easier that way to get the needed amount. Note: this will likely give you more gas and bloating, and more voluminous stools. If the gas and bloating do not go away in a few days, decrease the dosage. The reason I want you taking all that fiber is that, as your body starts dumping toxins, you must have fiber in your gut to take them out in the stool, or they will simply be reabsorbed into your system. The only contraindication is severe gastrointestinal disease, in which case you should, of course, consult with a doctor.

A 2013 study showed that consuming brassica-family foods results in lower rates of breast cancer.[21] Brassicas increase the activity of the crucial Phase I and Phase II liver enzymes, which I discuss in a later chapter (see page 162).

Eat lots of vegetables from the following list. While it's best to eat organically grown produce, the fruits and vegetables in the Clean 15 list aren't heavily sprayed. So, if you want to budget when to buy organically and when you can eat conventionally grown foods, base your choices on the Clean 15.

Clean 15

1. Avocado
2. Sweet corn*
3. Pineapples
4. Cabbage
5. Sweet peas

---

* Although sweet corn for human consumption is not currently a GMO food, with the increase in GMO agriculture, that may change.

6. Onions

7. Asparagus

8. Mangoes

9. Papayas

10. Kiwi fruit

11. Eggplant*

12. Grapefruit**

13. Cantaloupe (domestic)

14. Cauliflower

15. Sweet potatoes

About cooking on this plan: it's fine to cook your food, but be careful about frying or browning it. This way of cooking generates toxins you don't want right now. I recommend baking, braising, or steaming instead.

Eat Real, Unprocessed Food

Eat as many organically grown fruits and vegetables as you want, except tomato-family foods and grapefruit. Eat wild-caught small fish. Eat well-chewed nuts and seeds.

Use Turmeric but Not Pepper

Freely add spices like turmeric, but not black pepper or cayenne pepper. Turmeric is excellent for promoting liver detoxification and decreasing inflammation. Black pepper, however, increases gut permeability, which we do not want. And cayenne pepper, although it is a very healthy food, acts like members of the nightshade family of foods in slowing down some key liver-detoxification enzymes.

---

* Eggplant technically belongs to a family of foods called nightshades, which I advise you avoid on this diet. This group also includes potatoes, tomatoes, peppers, and tomatillos. Nightshades have been known to cause cartilage inflammation in some people. I have had a number of patients with osteo- and rheumatoid arthritis get better by avoiding nightshades.

** One food on the Clean 15 list that we need to eliminate, no matter how clean it is, is grapefruit. That is because grapefruit is unfortunately high in the bioflavonoid naringenin, which inhibits a key liver-detoxification enzyme.

Use Oils Carefully

Technically, oils are a refined food. Flax oil and fish oil are fine in moderation, but be sure they are toxin-free: fish oils can have a lot of POPs, which you are so diligently trying to get rid of. It's fine to cook with oils as long as the temperature is not too high. Once oils start to smoke, they are damaged and potentially toxic. If you're making a sauté, use water, and add the oil after the food is cooked.

The Maybes

The big "maybe" is coffee. Obviously, you should not be taking any sugar or milk in your coffee during these two weeks, but should you be drinking coffee at all? Coffee is unique in that it does upregulate some key detoxification enzymes and may actually increase glutathione levels. However, whether coffee works for you personally depends on whether you are able to detox the caffeine easily. This depends on your individual genetics. I have advised my patients in the past not to drink coffee during this important detoxification process. However, based on the recent research, I am reconsidering my position. I simply don't have enough new experiences with patients to make a clear recommendation.

After all the foods that this diet eliminates, you may be wondering whether there's anything left to eat. Trust me, there is! The daily portions of vegetables, especially brassicas, and the fiber supplements will leave you feeling full. And all that fiber will carry the toxins from your system.

Meal Plans for the Two-Week Diet

The meal plans for the Two-Week Diet are based on the Do's and Don'ts you've just read. Following this carefully thought-out meal plan will provide you with fourteen days of delicious and nourishing meals. This is the food that will support your detoxification. Feel free to modify and adapt these suggestions while staying within the basic guidelines.

Table 3.2. **Meal Plans for the Two-Week Diet**

DAY 1	
Breakfast	Zucchini omelet with sliced oranges
Midmorning snack	Dairy-free coconut yogurt with chopped almonds and berries
Lunch	Poached wild-caught cod with fennel and cauliflower
Midafternoon snack	Oven-baked organic kale chips with avocado dip
Dinner	Garlic broccoli with lamb chop and dairy-free Caesar salad
DAY 2	
Breakfast	Scrambled eggs with chopped Brussels sprouts
Midmorning snack	Organic strawberry smoothie with hemp milk
Lunch	Watercress and sunflower seed salad with sardines, organic kale chips
Midafternoon snack	Chia seed pudding
Dinner	Grilled vegetables with cauliflower "rice" and carrot-cabbage salad
DAY 3	
Breakfast	Pumpkin pecan soup
Midmorning snack	Organic apple with almond butter
Lunch	Curried egg salad with pea shoot salad and dilled broccoli and cauliflower
Midafternoon snack	Vegetable crudités with hummus
Dinner	Black bean and red quinoa soup, lamb burgers
DAY 4	
Breakfast	Energizing oatmeal with organic apples
Midmorning snack	Coconut kefir with berries
Lunch	Lentil burger with lemony slaw
Midafternoon snack	Carrots with chickpea dip
Dinner	Organic baked chicken, sweet potato, steamed broccoli, and green beans
DAY 5	
Breakfast	Deviled eggs with sesame green salad
Midmorning snack	Dairy-free yogurt with fruit and nuts
Lunch	Organic chicken salad with watercress and chopped steamed broccoli
Midafternoon snack	Lentil chips
Dinner	Braised wild-caught salmon, curried cauliflower and green bean sauté with dilled cucumber salad

DAY 6	
Breakfast	Dairy-free huevos rancheros with gluten-free tortilla
Midmorning snack	Baked peaches with nut crumble
Lunch	Hearty cabbage soup with gluten-free bread and almond butter
Midafternoon snack	Organic celery with sunflower-pecan spread
Dinner	Brassica stir-fry with wild salmon cakes
DAY 7	
Breakfast	Quinoa cereal with fresh fruit and dairy-free milk
Midmorning snack	Mocha hemp smoothie
Lunch	Lentil burgers with sesame green beans and napa cabbage salad
Midafternoon snack	Cilantro black bean soup
Dinner	Gluten-free quinoa spaghetti and grass-fed bison meatballs with tomato zucchini oreganata and tossed salad
DAY 8	
Breakfast	Hot amaranth cereal with pears and cashews, hemp milk
Midmorning snack	High-energy shake
Lunch	Black beans with mushroom gravy in baked sweet potato skins
Midafternoon snack	Cold cherry soup with coconut yogurt
Dinner	Roast turkey breast with braised Brussels sprouts, kasha, and cranberry-orange sauce
DAY 9	
Breakfast	Gluten-free coconut French toast topped with berries
Midmorning snack	Crudités with garlic nut dip
Lunch	Cold red-beet borscht and collard turkey roll-ups with sauerkraut
Midafternoon snack	Baked apple
Dinner	Baked cod with garlic string beans and sweet potato fries
DAY 10	
Breakfast	Cinnamon organic apple-nut porridge
Midmorning snack	Scoop of parsley/egg salad with chopped cucumber and celery
Lunch	Quinoa-stuffed acorn squash with turkey loaf
Midafternoon snack	Gluten-free bread with cashew nut butter
Dinner	Rosemary lamb chops with sautéed garlic broccoli and corn on the cob
DAY 11	
Breakfast	Organic spinach mushroom frittata with gluten-free bread
Midmorning snack	Green drink with spicy cashews

Lunch	Vegetable and bean chili with organic kale chips
Midafternoon snack	Gluten-free pear cobbler
Dinner	Stuffed sweet potatoes, green beans, and red cabbage slaw
DAY 12	
Breakfast	High-fiber cereal with berries
Midmorning snack	Walnuts with sliced organic apples
Lunch	Super-energy curried lentil soup with organic kale
Midafternoon snack	Homemade sweet potato chips
Dinner	White bean and cauliflower soup, baked wild-caught halibut with herbs and lentil salad
DAY 13	
Breakfast	Gluten-free waffles with berries
Midmorning snack	Protein smoothie with pectin
Lunch	Broccoli soup and Asian chopped organic chicken cabbage roll-ups
Midafternoon snack	Wheat-free pita triangles with hummus
Dinner	Black bean sesame loaf, grilled mushrooms, and sweet potatoes
DAY 14	
Breakfast	Eggs over easy with sautéed Swiss chard
Midmorning snack	Rainbow fruit salad
Lunch	Adzuki bean burger with stir-fried shiitake mushrooms and sauerkraut
Midafternoon snack	Organic popcorn with olive oil and nutritional yeast
Dinner	Curried lamb stew with lentils, cabbage, carrots, garlic, and parsley

What to Expect

During the first week you may be surprised by how you feel. You may feel light-headed, confused, tired, craving certain foods, and cranky, with an upset gut and especially bad breath. A lot is happening. You are:

- Withdrawing from foods and substances like sugar, salt, meat, gluten, and dairy, to which you are habituated or addicted.
- Changing the balance of bacteria in your gut, which means some bad bacteria are dying and releasing their toxins.

- Releasing toxins from your cells.
- Reestablishing healthier physiology.

Natural medicine doctors have known for centuries that as the body becomes healthier and recovers from chronic disease, acute symptoms increase—but this lasts for only a few days. In general, natural healers do not interpret most symptoms as signs of disease but as evidence of the body's efforts to heal. Symptoms can even become intense enough to be called a "healing crisis." As you follow this nutritional plan over these two weeks, the goal is not intense detox. Nevertheless, depending on your own degree of toxicity, if you have symptoms that don't resolve in a few days, back off the diet a bit, or see a natural medicine doctor to help you with the process.

The first week, you will likely start craving foods that you eat most often and consider your favorites.

The second week is more difficult to predict. Usually, you will start feeling quite a bit better since the initial intense toxin release and food withdrawal symptoms will have abated. People on this program often notice that their body is simply starting to work better again, and many people feel decades younger.

Is This Dangerous?

While this detox program is strenuous, it's safe—except in certain situations. What you undertake on this plan is far less strenuous than what our bodies can tolerate. Having helped a lot of patients detoxify, I have designed this program to minimize discomfort. Nonetheless, if you are seriously ill or feel that this is not working, by all means stop the protocol and see your doctor if needed. It's fine to be uncomfortable . . . it's not fine to injure yourself.

Note also that certain people should follow this protocol only under the supervision of a knowledgeable doctor. These include:

- Children

- People with type 1 diabetes

- Type 2 diabetics on insulin

- People whose blood sugar varies widely

- Patients with cancer

- People who are emaciated

Unfortunately, very few MDs are knowledgeable in this area. If you need support, I suggest you find a naturopathic doctor, broad-scope chiropractor, or MD certified in integrative or functional medicine.

Can I Just Keep Doing This Protocol?

Sorry, I realize you may now be quite excited by how much better you are feeling, but a detoxification diet is not the same as a healthy maintenance diet. The diet I have just presented is simply too low in protein to be optimal long-term. Nonetheless, there is no harm in continuing on it during the next two weeks as you do my Gut Cleanup Program in chapter 4. During chapter 5, "Restore Your Liver," and chapter 6, "Revive Your Kidneys," I will offer modified versions of this plan customized with special nutritional supports for those two detox organs.

To review: In these first two weeks, I am guiding you to rigorously stop putting toxins in your body. This is preparation for the next phase, in which you prepare your organs of elimination to get rid of toxins. Even though these first two weeks have only a limited goal—to simply decrease your intake of toxins—your body welcomes this so much that it begins its housecleaning. The first week may be tough, but by the second week the clear improvement in your health will make it all worthwhile. I know I am asking a lot of you, but fully engaging in my recommendations has a big payoff. You will feel healthier than you have in years—and we have only just begun your path to restoration.

4

Clean Up Your Gut

With each passing day, more and more people actively seek ways to detoxify. And that is due to increasing public concern about the mounting toxic load that contributes to symptoms and illness. I applaud this development! But knowing that detox is necessary is not the same as fully understanding *how* to safely detox. Nor does it mean that any and all detox approaches are equally effective. Or right for you. Yes, a quick detox might vastly improve your nutrition, compared with the stuff you were eating before. Yes, a daily diet of green drinks could work for you—if you are an eighteen- to twenty-five-year-old who's eaten clean foods since childhood, rarely drinks, and never smokes.

But what if you ate a lot of junk food as a child or during your teens? What if you were a party animal who drank and drugged your way through your teens and twenties?

What if in your thirties and forties you are a hardworking professional or a multitasking mom or dad who cuts corners to save time, gulping down a breakfast of doughnuts and coffee, eating takeout while working at your computer, guzzling sodas or downing protein bars to keep your energy going as you rush through the day and work on into the night?

What if, without knowing it, you were born with an underfunctioning detox capacity?

Or what if you have landed in your late forties or fifties with low energy, weight gain, fatigue, stress, anxiety, and poor sleep?

In all these extremely common scenarios—and notice that I don't even mention people who have joined the swelling ranks of those with chronic illnesses, chronic pain, or even more serious health conditions—you need a more highly calibrated form of detox. Healthy food and drink, while providing you with a sound nutritional baseline, cannot alone rectify the damage already done to your organs of detoxification over your lifetime.

Instead, it's essential that the organs of elimination themselves (gut, liver, and kidneys) first be repaired. And to ensure that you initiate detox safely, they must be repaired in the right sequence. Otherwise, you can unleash more toxins than your body can safely handle. Yes, you need to detox, but your body's detoxification organs need help—a lot of help—to detox effectively. And that's what the next three chapters will provide.

In chapter 2 of *The Toxin Solution,* you learned the simplest ways to decrease toxic load from all sources as much as possible, given that toxins are everywhere. Then, by following the Two-Week Jumpstart Diet, you further decreased toxins, while adding healthy nontoxic nutrition to give yourself a good baseline. The goal of this and the next two chapters is to introduce the right sequence of specific protocols to support each of the major detox organs—gut, liver, and kidney, in turn. As each organ is cleaned up via my two-week protocols, you can move on to the next. That way, you are encouraging toxins to leave your body in a way that your body can handle.

It Begins with the Gut

In this chapter, I begin with the gut and digestive tract, which is where detox must always start.

Why? Because unless you first clean up the gut, you keep passing along all of its toxins and toxic by-products to the next organ downline—the liver. A toxic gut, which constantly leaks poisonous metabolites and other noxious substances, overloads the liver and kidneys. Initiating detox without first repairing your gut is like going through your home emptying all the dirt, waste, and throwaways into one giant garbage bag and then emptying that garbage bag into your refrigerator. Unless you are ready to take that garbage out the back door to the refuse containers, the effort is pointless. While this may seem like an extreme comparison, it's not far off the mark. If your gut is overflowing with toxins it can't process, it will pass along all that garbage to other areas of your body, where it will undermine healthy function.

To prevent other detox organs from getting overwhelmed, before stirring up toxin release, you must first lower the toxic load in the gut. Following my program will do that. Otherwise, if you begin to detox before this preparation, the body will protest.

That is why in this chapter you will first ensure that your gut is in good shape. In later chapters, I will help you open up key detox pathways in your liver and kidneys.

Conrad's Story

Conrad's wife, Maryanne, practically dragged him into my office. I've seen this scenario dozens of times, since women are generally much more attentive to health than men. Conrad was embarrassed to speak about his primary problem. He, ahem, was "not taking care" of his wife in bed. He had lost interest and capacity. Maryanne (also a patient of mine) was not happy. Because Conrad was only forty-five years old, this should not have been a problem for them.

Conrad's diet was quite good, since Maryanne prepared their meals and had been following my nutritional guidance. (Though I suspect he regularly sneaked in unhealthy fast food.)

In a physical examination, I found nothing except for a tender and slightly enlarged liver. When I asked about Conrad's work environment, I learned that he was an expert in fiberglass-boat repair (another of my patients who worked on boats). Although he took appropriate exposure precautions, they were clearly inadequate. Fiberglass is composed of plastic reinforced by glass fibers. To repair a boat, Conrad had to first use liquid epoxies and resins on the boat surface, next position glass fiber sheets on the damaged area, and finally coat with glues and resins. As you can imagine, this process releases huge amounts of toxic chemicals. While the body can rid itself of some of these chemicals, the process uses up the stores of detox essentials, such as the master antioxidant, glutathione. With constant exposure to toxins, glutathione levels plummet and the detox process is weakened. The result is that the most harmful chemicals can build up in the body. What's more, a buildup of fiberglass dust is undesirable because it is carcinogenic.

To address Conrad's toxic load, I put him on my then-standard detoxification program—and learned a hard lesson. When he came back to see me the following week (this time without his wife), he was not doing well. Counter to my instructions, he had gone out for drinks a few times with his buddies and had sneaked a few smokes. Relapsing into his old habits in the midst of a rapid detox made him feel sick as a dog.

What happened? When in the midst of his detox, with toxic chemicals already being released from his fat stores, Conrad smoked and consumed alcoholic drinks. Instead of releasing toxins, he took in additional toxins. Aged beverages, like his favorite whiskey, contain multiple difficult-to-detoxify aldehydes, esters, and ketones. Detox system overload!

So what did we do? First, Conrad stopped the detox program at once. Next, I used the same methods I offer in chapters 5 and 6 to slow his rate of detox (take more fiber and consume more calories). Then I used the protocol in this chapter to prepare his gut, followed by the protocols in the next two chapters to prepare his liver and kidneys. Only after that preparation was Conrad ready to safely let go of all the toxins accumulated from his occupational exposures. After fully completing the Toxin

Solution, he was surprised he felt so much better—in all ways. Maryanne was happy again, too.

As you can see, the mistake I made with Conrad early in my professional career is the same one many people make when they initiate a detox program. To detoxify safely, you must balance the rate of toxin release with your ability to detoxify and excrete the toxins. The gut is a big source of toxins for most people. Following the advice in this and the next two chapters will save you from repeating that mistake.

Improving the function of the gut and downline detox organs is a lot easier once you slow the ongoing, daily barrage of toxins, as you have already started doing on this program. Nevertheless, toxicity will likely increase in your body—until you repair the leaky gut and eliminate all toxic gut bacteria, which is what you will do during week one of the Two-Week Gut Protocol in this chapter. My advice is: don't put this off to another day. The gut-detoxification protocol, which you will learn more about shortly, dramatically decreases the bad bacteria in your gut and improves gut integrity, so that any toxins produced in the gut are less able to circulate through your body.

Although it's now more widely recognized that the wrong gut bacteria contribute to increased disease risk, when I started seeing patients in 1973 this was essentially unknown. I was one of only two licensed male midwives in all of North America at the time, and most of my practice was helping women and young families. I noted that many women experienced vaginal and digestive upset after one to two weeks of taking broad-spectrum antibiotics. The problems were especially bad in those who had taken antibiotics for years to treat acne or chronic urinary-tract infections.

Although the health-conscious public now understands how to rebuild healthy gut flora through taking probiotics, at the time little was known about this. At first I recommended yogurt, which didn't help as much as I expected. Then I asked some of the women to bring me their empty yogurt containers so I could look at the labels, and saw that the commercial brands were using probiotic strains that were easy to manufacture and store in grocery stores—but not natural or clinically effective for humans. I next searched the local grocery and health-food stores for yogurts with the right strains, and recommended those to my patients. Although the results were better, they were still not good enough. Prescribed professional probiotic supplements worked a bit better but still did not resolve the problem.

I realized that just supplying a few strains of healthy bacteria was not enough to eliminate the toxic bacterial overgrowth bred by long-term antibiotic use. I then tried several other strategies for killing off the bad bacteria. To test the results, I used something called the Obermeyer test (also known as the Indican test), which measures intestinal toxicity produced by the wrong bacteria in the gut. I quickly found that almost all these patients had a heavy load of toxin-producing bacteria.

After seeing thousands of patients and testing the results, I gradually learned what worked and what didn't. By following the protocol in this chapter, people suffering from many different kinds of chronic disease have created the foundation for restoring their health. After all, if you can't digest your food, how can you get the nutrients you need? And if your gut is dumping toxins into your blood, how can your body possibly work very well?

The Two-Week Gut Protocol

What's going on in your gut? If you are like most people who come to my clinic, probably a whole lot more than you realize. Your gut is filled with bacteria, good and bad. Sometimes, even good gut bacteria release chemicals your body can't easily handle. But it's much worse when you eat unhealthy foods and have a gut overgrown with the wrong bacteria. Fast "foods," ersatz "foods," or sodas and sweets not only provide unwanted chemicals; they also promote the growth of the wrong bacteria. When the wrong gut bacteria digest food, these bacteria release toxic chemical by-products (called *endotoxins*) that add to your preexisting toxic load. Broadly defined, this umbrella term refers to any unwanted molecule coming from gut bacteria or food constituents that disrupts metabolism and winds up producing ill health and disease. (The strictest definition of "endotoxin" is bacterial-cell-wall-derived lipopolysaccharides. I prefer the broader definition above as more clinically relevant.) And aggravating these problems is a damaged, leaky gut.

Research shows that leaky gut is present in most chronic diseases, such as depression, diabetes, irritable bowel syndrome, inflammatory bowel disease, and rheumatoid arthritis. My best estimate is that one-third to one-half the North American population have excessive gut permeability. When the gut is leaky, undesirable food constituents and toxins from bacteria more easily enter your body.

These toxins inflame your gut and undermine gut function; but worse, they overload the liver and cause indiscriminate damage throughout the body. If you don't clean up the gut first, you will pass that toxic mess along to the liver, making its job of getting rid of toxic chemicals even tougher. That's why the goal of the program you will be following for the next two weeks is to:

1. Kill the bad bacteria in your gut.

2. Bind the toxic chemicals released as the bad bacteria die.

3. Reseed with good bacteria.

4. Repair your gut.

5. Stop the damage going forward.

As you will learn in this chapter, cleaning up gut toxins produces global health benefits. And throughout the rest of the chapter, I will give you a full picture of exactly how the science supports this assertion. You can get started by following this two-week protocol right away, as you continue reading this chapter. Each day, take all the recommended nutritional supplements and herbs. Read on after the protocol for a fuller explanation of how these recommendations will ready your gut to play its crucial role.

The good news is that there is a lot you can do to clean up the gut. And that is what you will do over the next two weeks through the protocols I offer in this chapter.

Table 4.1. **Two-Week Gut Detoxification and Improvement Protocol**

STEP		DAYS 1–7	DAYS 8–14
Step 1. Kill the bad bacteria	Fiber supplements, 2 grams three times per day	X	
	Goldenseal root powder, 1 teaspoon three times per day (six capsules)	X	
	Raw garlic cloves, two cloves per day	X	
Step 2. Repair the gut	Multibacterial probiotic that includes *Lactobacillus* and especially *Bifidobacterium* strains, one capsule three times per day	X	X
	Fresh cabbage juice, 1 quart per day		X
	Quercetin, 250 mg two times per day		X
	DGL, 250–500 mg three times per day, letting lozenges dissolve in the mouth		X

The Gut and Toxicity

Many people don't like to think about what goes on "down there" and assume that our digestive systems can handle anything we eat—until symptoms say otherwise.

When I was a third-year naturopathic medical student, my professor, Robert Carroll, DC, ND, started the first class of the year with the provocative statement "Death begins in the colon!" This statement contradicted what I had learned in my two years of basic science courses. The textbooks I studied in those courses contended that the gut was a long tube, covered with a perfect protective membrane that admitted only nutrients the body needed while effectively keeping out the "wrong" bacteria and their toxic after-products. Medical wisdom of that time held that the gut was completely impermeable to anything bad. Today, the wide prevalence of "leaky gut" reveals how naive that notion was. But back then, few understood this.

I was therefore surprised to hear Professor Carroll's claim that the digestive as well as many other health problems that so many people experienced resulted from gut toxicity. Restoring the gut to health and strengthening digestion improve overall health dramatically, he said. Later, as a medical student, when I went on clinical rounds I saw how common gut problems are in people suffering from a wide range of diseases. Still, I remained skeptical about the connection between the gut, toxicity, and health—until I began practicing on my own.

What Goes On in a Toxic Gut?

As I discussed earlier, the primary sources of external toxins are the foods you eat, the lotions and potions you put on your skin, and the chemicals you use to clean your home and care for your garden. However, another very important source of toxins arises from *within* your body—specifically, from your gut. Technically, the gut—a long tube coiled up in the abdomen, with the mouth at one end and the anus at the other—is actually "outside" the body. Open at both ends, the gut, unlike the rest of the body, is a nonsterile environment, full of bacteria. In fact, there are ten times as many bacteria in your gut as there are cells in your body. Every single day, those bacteria actively produce a lot of metabolites.

Understanding Metabolites

Metabolites are small molecules that are involved in almost all of the body's metabolic processes. Nearly every physiological function, including energy production, is part of an ongoing chain of activities. The small molecules called *metabolites* either contribute to, or result from, these activities. But if they are the wrong metabolites, from bad bacteria, they can also poison these life-dependent metabolic processes. I mention this because I use the term *metabolite* quite frequently. Understanding this is highly relevant to detox. Why? Because health is all about optimizing the balance of molecules, metabolites, and enzyme functions in the body.

For this to happen, the critically needed nutrients have to be absorbed from the gut; detox, on the other hand, entails processing the harmful molecules and metabolites *out* of your system in a way that ensures that they do the least damage. For example, clostridia are bad bacteria that produce highly toxic metabolites that are easily absorbed into the body when the gut membrane's integrity is damaged.

Bacteria and the Gut

If you have good bacteria in your system, these will produce welcome molecules like B vitamins. But if you have the wrong bacteria, they will produce noxious endotoxin metabolites, with names like *indoles* and *skatoles,* that circulate in your system, disrupting metabolism. Although these terms have little meaning to the average person, what if I tell you that indoles and skatoles are also called *cadaverine* and *putrescine,* respectively? Does that begin to give you an idea of why you don't want them? As these names imply, these are metabolites produced during decay.

In my first year as a primary-care naturopathic doctor, during the occasionally slow days of building my practice, I voraciously read medical journals. To my great surprise, one day I read a startling and controversial study reporting that, even in healthy humans, up to 1 percent of ingested proteins are absorbed *intact* through the intestinal wall—directly contradicting what I had just learned in the standard medical physiology textbooks. Instead of fully digesting the food, the gut allows a very small amount of food proteins, other molecules, and even bacteria to enter the body without being broken down. Hmm, that didn't sound like an impermeable gut to me. In fact, the body is constantly intentionally sampling the contents of the gut so it can be on guard against infectious organisms. The gut has to be very smart, welcoming in all the needed nutrients, keeping out all the toxins, while carefully letting through a tiny bit of everything so it can protect against infection.

Absorption of any more than a tiny amount signifies that there are gaps in your gut wall and the body is losing control. Just like holes in a wall, these gaps indiscriminately let stuff in. They undermine gut integrity. Just as a balloon with pinprick holes on its surface can't contain air, a damaged gut cell wall can't contain the gut bacteria and toxins and keep them from entering your bloodstream. And once in the bloodstream, undigested food molecules can stimulate allergies and other immune reactions.

But that's not all. The study also revealed that the absorption rate of intact proteins increases to as much as 10 percent during severe gastro-intestinal infection when the gut lining is seriously damaged. That was the first solid research I read on how gut imbalances and gut permeability profoundly impact health. The vital importance of a well-functioning gut is better understood nowadays. Today's integrative medicine clinicians know that gut issues like maldigestion, malabsorption, leaky gut, and harmful bacteria contribute to, and may even cause, most chronic diseases.

Jane's Story

At age thirty-two, Jane had been recently diagnosed as having the early stages of rheumatoid arthritis. Although her morning pain and stiffness weren't too bad and easily relieved by two aspirin, she was quite dis-traught. Her mother and all her aunts suffered from severe forms of the disease, so badly in some cases that their hands were quite deformed. She was not willing to accept her family physician's prognosis that she was fated to live with a disease that would relentlessly progress despite multiple drugs.

Fortunately, she came to see me before her disease had progressed very far. I explained to her that I thought her joint inflammation was being caused by the triple whammy of a leaky gut (due to food allergies), toxic gut bacteria, and overreactive inflammatory activity. (Inflammation is a normal, important process in our body that replaces damaged tissues and fights infection. Unfortunately, modern lifestyle and diet result in overactivation of this process.) While all of this was new to her, she was eager to do whatever was necessary. Since many people are allergic to wheat and dairy, I suggested that she eliminate them from her diet.

She followed a diet, like the one on this program, that minimized toxins. It consisted of fish, fruits, vegetables, beans, nuts, and seeds. She also took the supplements I recommend for gut cleanup.

By the end of two weeks, her symptoms had already decreased by 50 percent. After one month of carefully following this diet-and-supplement prescription, she had no further pain in her joints. After three months, all her lab-test levels had returned to normal!

Not all of my rheumatoid arthritis patients respond so well. I still vividly remember with great sadness a fifty-five-year-old woman who had had the disease for over twenty years. Her hands were so deformed she could hardly hold a pen, and she was having chronic stomach problems from all the aspirin and other drugs she was taking. Although I applied exactly the same therapy, all we could accomplish was lowering her drug dosage. Sometimes diseases do progress to cause such serious damage, that they are past the body's ability to heal.

Although people often can heal even supposedly "incurable" diseases, it's important to act promptly rather than wait too long. The earlier an underlying problem is corrected, the better the outcome.

The gut is one of the hardest-working systems in the body. It has the very challenging job of digesting food—absorbing the nutrients from the food but not the toxins released by bacteria in our gut—while activating the immune system to kill the harmful bacteria off without damaging the desirable bacteria. Turns out the gut is actually pretty smart, maintaining careful control of what is allowed into the body, and what is kept out and then excreted in the stools.

Understanding the Gut Protocol

As you can see, restoring your gut confers many benefits. It will set the stage for detox, and it will help you recover and prevent many other illnesses. In undertaking this protocol, you can also rely on the good results experienced by hundreds of my patients. No one has ever been hurt by it, while many have been grateful to finally get their health back. The results are quite remarkable. Everyone reports simply feeling healthier. The basic approach is to:

- Kill off the toxic bacteria.

- Bind the toxins released from the bad bacteria as they die.

- Recolonize the intestines with good bacteria.

- Use herbs and nutrients to promote healing of the damaged gut cells.

The first step is getting the right nutritional baseline. Following the Two-Week Jumpstart Diet gives you everything you need. The foods and meal plans are high in flavonoids, carotenoids, and fiber to help you decrease gut permeability. Included are a rainbow of healthy fruits and vegetables that will help you safely release gut toxins, decrease inflammation, and make healthy molecules like butyric acid, which promotes intestinal-cell health.[1] I suggest that you continue following the diet I recommended in chapter 3 for these next two weeks, while implementing the Two-Week Gut Protocol. At the end of this chapter, I'll let you know what to avoid going forward to preserve your newly re-created gut health.

Week 3: Step 1. Kill the Bad Bacteria

For three days before starting this program, take fiber supplements, using 2 grams of fiber three times a day. As I mentioned earlier, the fiber helps ensure the prompt excretion of toxic bacteria via the stools.

Beginning on day 1, and for the next seven days, take 1 teaspoonful (six capsules) of goldenseal root powder (*Hydrastis canadensis*) three times a day. This great herbal medicine kills the harmful bacteria in your gut while being friendly to the healthy bacteria. You can also eat raw garlic if you want to speed up the process, since this interesting vegetable is also good at killing the bad bacteria. (However, please don't visit me!) About 5 percent of the population, like me, have difficulty detoxifying the complex sulfur compounds found in raw garlic and, to a lesser extent, in other members of the onion (genus *Allium*) family. While I have never had a patient report problems with this protocol, if it makes you feel unwell, please make sure to slow down the process by taking less goldenseal and garlic, but definitely do not decrease the fiber. Though initially taking fiber may cause you to experience more intestinal gas, your body will adapt within a few days. Be sure to drink plenty of water with the fiber.

Week 4: Step 2. Repair the Gut

Now that you have eliminated the toxic bacteria, you will recolonize the gut with optimal bacteria. Three times per day, outside of mealtimes, take a good-quality multi-bacterial-strain probiotic (one that includes ten or more types of bacteria) with several species of *Lactobacillus* and, especially, of *Bifidobacterium*. This latter organism is one of the most researched, showing health benefits in many areas. Most health-food stores have several good options. (Good to take probiotics in Week 3 as well.)

Healing the Gut Walls

After you get rid of the bad bacteria in your gut, you can take various foods, nutrients, and herbs to facilitate regeneration of the gut cells.

Cabbage-family foods are high in glutamine, a healing nutrient that helps repair the gut walls. Cabbage also contains sulforaphanes, which increase liver detoxification. Drinking one quart a day of the fresh cabbage (or sauerkraut) juice is so powerful, it even heals stomach ulcers. You can get bottled cabbage juice, but the best way to obtain it is to make your own using a juicer. Add one beet and two stalks of celery to one-quarter head of cabbage to make a half quart of cabbage juice. I prefer juicers that keep the fiber in the juice—and they are also easier to clean. Even if, like some people, you decide you really like the taste, I strongly advise that you only drink this amount of cabbage juice for the time that I recommend here. Cabbage has compounds that bind iodine in the gut. This is not a problem in the short term, but after a few months it can decrease iodine levels (which are already low in the majority of the population) and cause a lower level of thyroid hormone production.

If you are among the group who don't like the smell or taste of cabbage juice, you can take glutamine,[2] one of the key, gut-healing nutrients in cabbage, 500 mg, three times per day. I always prefer to use food whenever possible, so try the juice first: you may be amazed at how much you come to enjoy it. Surprisingly, gut regeneration doesn't take long; it can be accomplished in the one week you will do this program—as long as you also stop damaging the gut as discussed below.

Taking 250 mg of quercetin twice a day helps quench inflammatory processes in the gut. If you want to obtain quercetin from a food source instead, add yellow onions to your diet. Quercetin is what gives them their yellow color.[3]

I recommend taking licorice in the form of DGL (deglycyrrhizinated licorice), 250 to 500 mg, three times a day, letting the lozenges dissolve in your mouth. Researchers have documented for decades the power of licorice root to heal the digestive system's damaged mucous membranes. One study found a 52 percent reduction in symptoms using licorice compared with 24 percent in those receiving a sugar-candy placebo.[4]

Licorice is particularly effective for healing stomach ulcers and the mucosal damage caused by aspirin, as mentioned below.[5] You can use cabbage and yellow onions or glutamine and quercetin supplements for as long as you want, but licorice can be used for only a few months, because some people develop high blood pressure from it. That's why I prefer DGL, another form of licorice, which has the problematic blood-pressure molecule removed and can be taken as long as you want.

Licorice and "Singer's Voice"

My late teacher Dr. John Bastyr, after whom I named Bastyr University, was for decades the favorite doctor of the Seattle Opera. When performers from that troupe suffered from "singer's voice" and became too hoarse to perform, they turned to him, because his "secret" herb (licorice) was so effective. Because I now lecture so much internationally on toxicity and detoxification, I have learned to always have licorice fluid extract (more concentrated than the tincture) with me: as my voice starts to fade after three to four hours of lecturing, I can always count on it to give me another hour or two of voice.

As the gut heals, your health is radically improved.

- You reduce the amount of endotoxins in your blood.

- Inflammation calms down.

- You can absorb nutrients from food.

- Your gut cells now keep in the gut what belongs in the gut, protecting the rest of your body.

- You are prepared to successfully detox.

All of these benefits await you, and to ensure that you are motivated, I want to reveal all that goes into an unhealthy gut—and it's quite a lot!

The Dangers of an Unhealthy Gut

Why does *The Toxin Solution* emphasize gut health to the extent of devoting two full weeks to it? Because when the digestion is not working properly, the gut becomes too permeable—or, in common parlance, "leaky." When the gut "leaks," undesirable molecules, food antigens, bacteria cell parts, and so on get through the gut membrane. Leaky gut syndrome triggers many other undesirable biochemical activities. For example, instead of keeping allergic substances and other toxins confined to the gut, a permeable gut-cell lining allows these to circulate through the body.

Since human gut contents can be either beneficial or problematic, Mother Nature wisely designed our bodies so that all the blood from the gut first goes through the liver, to be detoxified before it circulates through the bloodstream. The bad news is that when this process goes awry—with bad gut flora, leaky gut, and liver dysfunction (all extremely common)—this toxic mess ends up overwhelming the liver and entering the body. Although leaky gut therefore contributes to most chronic disease, you don't have to have a diagnosed serious disease to be suffering damage from a leaky gut.

For all of these reasons, the condition of your gut is a primary factor in your health. Unfortunately, few doctors understand and use this key insight. And yet, research connects endotoxins with diabetes, heart disease, and mitochondrial damage, among other problems. For example, a research group in Germany followed 122 patients with chronic cardiac failure—an advanced case of heart disease. They found that after two years, those with the highest level of endotoxins had a dramatically higher rate of death, with one-half the patients dying.[6] In other words, endotoxins contribute to—and compound—a wide range of health issues.

The two main problems with endotoxins are that they:

- Contribute to toxic overload.

- Prevent your body from detoxifying successfully.

There is still some debate about the primary mechanisms. The body contains around ten pounds of gut bacteria—there are ten times more bacteria than there are cells of the body. Some bacterial metabolites may be beneficial. Endotoxins clearly are not. One theory holds that gut endotoxins use up liver capacity so that there is less ability to detox other poisons. Another possible scenario is that fat buildup in the liver (due to endotoxins) causes progressive dysfunction such that the liver can less effectively detoxify the gut toxins, thus allowing more of them to pass into circulation. When left unchecked, these toxic gut chemicals increase damaging oxidative stress throughout the body. Whether either or both theories turn out to be most accurate, it's best to address endotoxins.

How Gut Toxins Cause Specific Diseases

In this section, I will help you understand what the Two-Week Gut Protocol is designed to correct. Let's first highlight just a few of the ways in which the wrong bacteria in your gut cause toxicity and damage, including the following:

- Production of inflammatory chemicals, which translates into increased risk for cardiovascular illness, diabetes, and other health concerns.
- Conversion of nutrients to toxins, so that you are both nutritionally deprived *and* toxic.
- Conversion of dietary polysaccharides to sugar, which results in increased absorption of sugar and increased production of fat from carbohydrates—all of which contribute to weight gain and diabetes. Obese people convert polysaccharides to sugar at a much higher rate than lean people due to the types of bacteria present in their guts.
- Poisoning of mitochondria, which support health and vitality. Twenty-five percent of the volume of the typical cell consists of mitochondria.
- Undermining of the liver's detoxification processes.

Gut toxins are also responsible for weight gain, obesity, and diabetes. If you have ever tried to diet, it's important to understand this. Even if you carefully avoid sugar, the wrong gut bacteria will convert healthy complex carbohydrates, like those found in beans, potatoes, and pasta, to simple sugars, the same types of carbs found in sweets. Intriguing new research shows that obese people actually lose weight when given bacteria extracted from the guts of lean people—with no change in diet. Of course, if the obese people stay on their unhealthy diet, they will stimulate the regrowth of the same toxic bacteria.

Here's another key finding: the higher the endotoxin level, the higher the insulin resistance. In insulin resistance, a precursor to diabetes, the body's cells do not respond to the presence of insulin. As a result, insulin can't do its job of getting sugar from the bloodstream into the cells so it can be converted into energy and instead is stored in fat. People with the highest levels of gut endotoxins (the top 25 percent) have a greater than threefold increased risk of diabetes, compared with those in the bottom 25 percent.[7]

In addition, as endotoxins increase, levels of the good HDL cholesterol go down.[8] This leads to increased toxic overload. Why? Because HDL is the "garbage truck" that carries endotoxins to the liver for elimination. HDL also carries fat-soluble toxins—like the POPs mentioned in chapters 1 and 2—to the liver for detoxification. So the endotoxins act as a double whammy: they are directly toxic, and they make it more difficult to get rid of other toxins by filling up the HDL, which is then unable to transport them to the liver. One reason why people with high HDL levels have less heart disease may simply be that they are better able to get rid of the highly inflammatory endotoxins.

What's worse is that the wrong gut bacteria can change normal, healthy food constituents into toxins. For example, the wrong bacteria convert choline—which you need for cell membranes and neurotransmitters—into the toxic compound trimethylamine (TMA), which in turn is rapidly converted to trimethylamine-N-oxide (TMAO). TMAO results in the accumulation of cholesterol, causing atherosclerosis (plaque in the arteries).[9]

And that's not all. The wrong gut bacteria make people reabsorb the very toxins the liver works so hard to release! Here's how: In a process called Phase II liver detoxification, the body excretes chemical toxins by

Figure 4.1. **Conversion of dietary choline to toxic TMA by inappropriate gut flora**

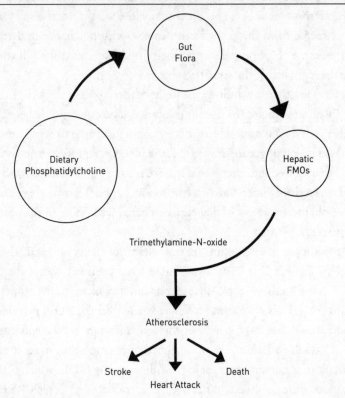

binding them, through a process called *conjugation,* to other molecules that safely carry them through the bile and into the gut, where they are eventually excreted (or to the kidneys for elimination in the urine). But when you have the wrong bacteria and not enough fiber, the bacteria remove the conjugating molecule—the molecule that makes the substance nontoxic—leading to the toxins' reabsorption. This is why almost everyone is toxic: when you eat too little fiber and have the wrong gut bacteria, you lack the ability to get toxins out of the body.

Figure 4.1 source: W. H. Tang, Z. Wang, B. S. Levison, et al., "Intestinal microbial metabolism of phosphatidylcholine and cardiovascular risk," *New England Journal of Medicine* 368, no. 17 (2013): 1575–84.

For all these reasons, eliminating endotoxins through the protocol in this chapter will prevent many different kinds of illnesses, improve your nutrition, and set you up for healthy detoxification.

The Heart and Blood Sugar

Research also connects endotoxins with heart disease. As endotoxin levels rise, so do all the indicators of cardiovascular conditions—such as waist size, waist–hip ratio, total cholesterol, serum triglycerides, serum insulin levels, and other health problems. These markers also signify increased inflammation throughout the body. The immune system is always on alert to defeat an invading virus, bacterium, or fungus. This is an important way the body protects us from infection and regenerates tissues. But when inflammation is chronic, the immune system is overactivated, causing unintentional tissue damage. This is a key reason that most diseases, especially chronic diseases, derive from excessive

Figure 4.2. **How gut endotoxins disrupt metabolism**

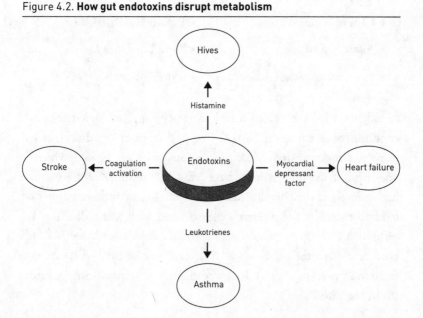

inflammation. And it is also why so many disease names end in *-itis* (a suffix denoting diseases characterized by inflammation)—rheumatoid arthritis, osteoarthritis, dermatitis, and so on. But many other diseases also have a strong inflammatory component—for example, asthma, atherosclerosis, and Alzheimer's disease.

Healing your gut is a must, because almost everyone with any type of chronic disease has a leaky gut. The conditions that are most closely linked to leaky gut are:

- Abdominal bloating
- Aphthous stomatitis
- Asthma
- Atopic dermatitis
- *Blastocystis hominis*
- *Candida albicans*
- Celiac disease
- Chronic stress
- *Entamoeba histolytica*
- Essential fatty acid deficiency
- Food allergies
- Giardia
- Hypochlorhydria
- Inflammatory bowel disease
- Irritable bowel syndrome
- Migraine
- Psoriasis
- Rheumatoid arthritis
- Type 1 diabetes
- Type 2 diabetes

When the levels of toxins from leaky gut get high enough, the health condition worsens even further—to a dangerous condition called *metabolic endotoxemia* (ME). Most people who are obese—which is one-third of the population—have ME. This means they have much higher levels of the chemicals that produce chronic inflammation and oxidative stress.[10] ME is strongly associated with many diseases. It's unknown how many people in the general population have ME. It's present in diabetes, cardiovascular disease, and obesity—I'd estimate in 10 to 25 percent of cases. It can be diagnosed by measuring endotoxins in the blood.

John's Story

John was sick all the time, feeling like he always had the flu. He had recently read an article about "hidden infections" and thought an undiagnosed viral infection was causing his problems. When he came into my office, his problem seemed pretty obvious, since this five-foot-eight-inch man weighed about 275 pounds. Nonetheless, because I wanted to be supportive of his taking control of his health, I drew several vials of blood and sent them to the lab for every then-available test for infection. All the results were negative for acute or chronic infection.

I gave him an Indican test (a urine test that measures toxins that come from the gut). The results indicated a lot of gut toxicity. I explained to him that a toxic gut produces many of the same inflammatory molecules released when we have a viral infection and that he likely had ME. John assumed that I would, like other doctors, simply tell him to lose weight. I surprised him by explaining that his toxic gut was far worse for his health than being overweight.

John immediately started on the gut-detoxification program. Every two weeks we reran his Indican test, and as his toxicity decreased, so, too, did his symptoms. After six months, his Indican test was normal and all his symptoms were gone. He had also lost twenty pounds—without trying to lose weight! As you'd expect, he was very happy with the results.

Diseases Associated with Metabolic Endotoxemia[11]

- Cardiovascular disease
- Chronic inflammation
- Diabetes (type 2)
- Dyslipidemia
- Insulin resistance
- Nonalcoholic fatty liver disease (NAFLD)
- Obesity
- Stroke

Most people would be surprised to hear that the normally strong relationship between obesity and diabetes disappears when a person has a low level of toxicity. And overweight individuals who regularly exercise do not have the expected increase in heart disease. I am not saying that obesity is good for you! What I am saying is that the toxicity and lack of exercise that typically *cause* the obesity are the problem. Decreasing toxins and engaging in healthy behaviors are more important than what the scale says.

As John's case reveals, a toxic gut is worse than merely being overweight. Even if you don't have full-blown ME, endotoxins send health in the wrong direction and increase the risk of getting these—and other—ailments. That is why it's vital to repair your gut and address endotoxins now.

(As an aside, one of the challenges in medicine is the constant fads. Back in the 1980s, "hidden infections" were the rage, and a number of chronically ill patients sought my help in diagnosing them. With only two exceptions, every one of them was suffering from an unhealthy diet and lifestyle, not a hidden infection.)

The source of many common ailments is not always intuitively obvious when symptoms manifest themselves. And that is one of the reasons why, in this book, I provide a lot of scientific background to help you feel confident in following my suggestions. It's important to both follow the program and understand *why* you are following the program. And it's also extremely important, once you have completed these two weeks, to avoid disrupting your gut going forward.

Stop the Damage Going Forward

Now that you have repaired the past damage to your gut, you may be wondering how to stop future damage. What undermines gut integrity? Good question! Let me single out four of the most important things to avoid if you want a healthy gut:

1. Nonsteroidal anti-inflammatory drugs

2. Excessive consumption of alcohol

3. Consumption of high-fructose corn syrup

4. Food allergies (discussed in chapter 7)

Though widely ingested, each of these attacks cell-wall integrity. Let's find out how they do this.

Nonsteroidal Anti-inflammatory Drugs

Aspirin and acetaminophen are the quintessential over-the-counter pain-management offerings. You may have heard the scientific term for them, which is *nonsteroidal anti-inflammatory drugs* (NSAIDs). (Yes, acetaminophen is not technically an NSAID, but they are typically grouped together.) Though convenient, and in wide use, these drugs cause far more harm than most doctors and users of them realize. Studies show that NSAIDs produce gut damage and gut permeability.[12] Thirty million people take NSAIDs every day. When taken regularly, it's been shown, NSAIDs both *increase* absorption of toxins and *decrease* absorption of the healthy nutrients your body gets from food—exactly

Table 4.2. **Gut Damage from Regular Use of NSAIDs**

ADVERSE EFFECT	FREQUENCY
Gut inflammation	60–70%
Leaky gut	44–70%
Malabsorption	40–70%
Mucosal ulceration	30–40%
Blood loss and anemia	30%

Table 4.2 source: C. Sostres, C. J. Gargallo, and A. Lanas, "Nonsteroidal anti-inflammatory drugs and upper and lower gastrointestinal mucosal damage," *Arthritis Research & Therapy* 15, suppl. 3 (2013): S3.

the opposite of what you want. Instead of using NSAIDs to dial down your perception of pain and other symptoms, it's far better to find and treat the causes of your symptoms. *All* NSAIDs increase gut permeability within hours of ingestion. NSAID-induced damage is estimated to significantly increase rate of death in users.

Other NSAIDs that increase gut permeability include ibuprofen, indomethacin, naproxen, Vioxx, and Feldene. I always recommend treating the causes, not the symptoms. Sometimes, of course, we need to decrease symptoms in the short run to allow time for healing to take place. But even then, I try to use natural therapies that support the body's own efforts to heal rather than drugs that are yet another chemical that the body has to detoxify. For example, women having menstrual cramps will often find magnesium with pyridoxal-5-phosphate (P5P) supplements more effective than NSAIDs. This also helps those suffering migraine. If you have an inflammatory condition like allergies or asthma along with migraine, you'll find the herb butterbur very helpful. Readers wanting to learn more about natural therapies for common diseases will find my *Encyclopedia of Natural Medicine* a helpful resource.

Excessive Consumption of Alcohol

In my early years as an extremely health-conscious new naturopathic doctor, I carefully avoided alcohol. My grandfather pointed out that all my long-lived forebears drank one or two full glasses of red wine every evening. I, of course, confident in my arrogance, was sure he was wrong. Well, wise sayings of yore endure because they contain a kernel of truth.

Let's look at what alcohol does to gut permeability. The more alcohol a person drinks, the leakier the gut. Note in figure 4.3 that even three hours after alcohol consumption, excessive gut permeability persists.

When alcohol meets your gut cells, it activates an enzyme called cytochrome P450 2E1 (CYP2E1), which detoxifies the alcohol. This process releases free radicals, which can be neutralized by glutathione, a major

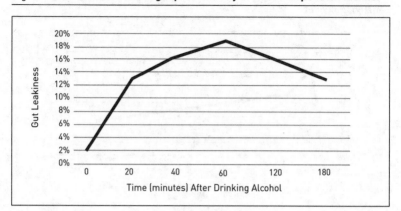

Figure 4.3. **Alcohol increases gut permeability in a dose-dependent manner**

antioxidant. But that can happen only if there's enough glutathione available. Once glutathione gets depleted by alcohol consumption, the free radicals multiply and alcohol leaks into the body.

When intestinal cells are damaged by alcohol, they also allow increased entry of endotoxins. In fact, some researchers now suggest that anxiety, depression, dementia, facial rash, and other symptoms associated with alcoholism may result from endotoxin damage, not just alcohol.

The research clearly shows that light to moderate alcohol consumption is healthful, while too much alcohol is quite damaging. But what constitutes healthful levels? The answer varies widely, based on genetics, nutritional status, and environmental toxin load.

For example, people deficient in vitamin D experience more leaky gut after consuming alcohol than those with adequate vitamin D levels. The majority of Americans are deficient in vitamin D. This deficiency makes gut permeability from other causes worse as well.

Bottom line: the safest approach is to follow the general guidelines of one or two alcoholic drinks per day for women and two or three per day for men.

Figure 4.3 source: Y. Wang, J. Tong, B. Chang, B. Wang, D. Zhang, and B. Wang, "Effects of alcohol on intestinal epithelial barrier permeability and expression of tight junction–associated proteins," *Molecular Medicine Reports* 9, no. 6 (2014): 2352–56.

Figure 4.4. **Alcohol causes release of free radicals in intestinal cells, causing leaky gut**

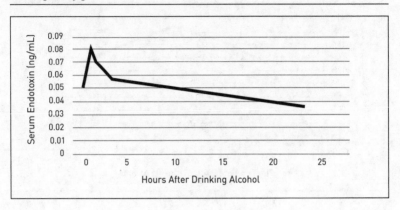

High-Fructose Corn Syrup

It used to be that only late-stage alcoholics suffered from fatty liver disease. But now *nonalcoholic* fatty liver disease (NAFLD) affects a stunning 31 percent of the U.S. population.[13] (It was 18 percent in 1990 and 29 percent in 2000.) Even children now suffer from this terrible illness. Children with NAFLD have ten times more endotoxins than healthy children.[14] The question is *why?*

It turns out that a few years before NAFLD was first seen, high-fructose corn syrup was introduced into our diets. Along with its well-known disruptive effects on blood-sugar regulation, high-fructose corn syrup (HFCS) raises endotoxin levels. Serious research now connects consumption of HFCS soft drinks and NAFLD.[15] In figure 4.5 you can see that the number of soft drinks consumed correlates with higher levels of fatty liver disease and metabolic syndrome (MS). When fed to mice at levels now commonly consumed by foolish humans, HFCS causes an elevation of endotoxins in the blood and outright NAFLD.[16]

Figure 4.4 source: S. Bala, M. Marcos, A. Gattu, D. Catalano, and G. Szabo, "Acute binge drinking increases serum endotoxin and bacterial DNA levels in healthy individuals," *PLoS One* 9, no. 5 (2014): e96864.

Figure 4.5. **Correlation between soft-drink consumption per day and fatty liver disease**

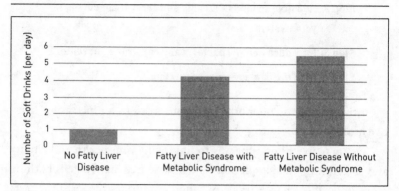

Going forward, to protect your healed gut from further damage, make sure to avoid consuming HFCS. It is not necessary to avoid fruit, which has fructose. The level of fructose in food is much lower than that found in soft drinks, and fructose in food is more slowly absorbed.

Food Allergens

Any kind of allergic response can cause gut-wall inflammation and leaky gut, increasing your risk for illness.

Conclusion

As you focus on healing the first pathway of detoxification—the gut and digestive function—you will accrue tremendous benefits. With a deeper understanding of the damage caused by a toxic gut, you can follow the four steps you need to take to heal it. To summarize:

Figure 4.5 source: W. Nseir, F. Nassar, and N. Assy, "Soft drinks consumption and nonalcoholic fatty liver disease," *World Journal of Gastroenterology* 16, no. 21 (2010): 2579–88.

Step 1. Eliminate the bad bacteria.

Step 2. Add fiber to bind the toxins and carry them out of your system.

Step 3. Introduce healthy bacteria and repair the gut walls.

Step 4. Stop the damage from recurring.

In chapter 7, I will offer other recommendations for increasing digestive health going forward.

You are now well on your way to improving your health and vitality and establishing the foundation for a disease-free life. There is nothing more important than a properly functioning intestine. Health starts with a clean gut with the right bacteria, well-functioning membranes, and effective digestion that completely breaks down foods so their life-dependent nutrients can be absorbed and toxins kept out.

As the gut heals, everything else gets better. And I truly mean *everything*. Endotoxins no longer poison you. Inflammation is calmed. The liver is no longer overloaded, so it can deal with the rest of the toxins. Nutrients can be better absorbed. All of this because the gut now works as it is supposed to.

Now, let's get your next key detoxification organs—your liver and kidneys—healed and functioning, and able to detoxify successfully.

5

Restore Your Liver

Before we proceed, let me congratulate you for coming this far. At this point, having a solid nutritional base and a better-functioning digestive system, many of you will feel noticeably better than you have in years, with more energy and stamina, and a lessening of most symptoms. It is from this place of well-being that your body is becoming ready to release the toxic load that is burdening you. If you are *not* noticing improvement, it may be for one of the following reasons:

1. Your health is already pretty good, and the improvement is subtle.

2. You have a weakened detox capacity, and your toxic load may already be compromising your health—an issue that this next two-week protocol will address.

3. You have been suffering from other health complaints and may benefit from the additional health supports found in this chapter.

If it's reason number 2, then I want to assure you that this phase of the program will make a real difference. If it's number 3, in addition to the regular protocol, which everyone can follow, later in this chapter I will provide some additional tips for making the protocol even more effective. (Of course, all of you health mavens who seek exceptional health can choose to use these enhancements as well.)

Now that we are at the halfway point, I strongly applaud you for following the program so far. And I also want to thank you for being one of the millions of people who are listening to their bodies and doing the right things for it. I know it isn't easy because there are so many loud voices out there "debunking" detox, as well as a lot of uninformed pooh-poohing of most natural and holistic therapies. But I hope that, by now, the benefits you have already experienced will give you confidence to begin active detox.

Before proceeding, I want to alert you that it's possible you will experience some minor symptoms during the next phase of the program. With active detox, you must prepare in two ways: physically and psychologically.

Physically, it's vital that you listen to your body and adjust the rate of your detox accordingly. After the protocol section, I will show you exactly how to do that.

Psychologically, you need to be prepared as well. It's normal during any detox to experience some minor reactions at first, such as fatigue, headaches, and other signs that I will explain more fully later. When people feel below par, that's often the time that their well-intentioned loved ones and friends rush in to question their decision to detoxify. "Why put yourself through this?" people may ask out of concern.

That's why I am offering a little pep talk here: so other people's lack of in-depth health knowledge won't undermine your motivation to heal yourself. As a result of a public campaign of ignorance, many doctors—and, as a result, many people—don't understand why the body needs support for detoxification.

The sad fact is that when people don't support their bodies' functional systems, whether it is the detox organs (which this book covers) or other organs, these systems will often wind up functioning below par—or malfunctioning altogether. People don't wind up with kidney failure or on kidney dialysis—to use an extreme example—because their organs and systems were working perfectly up until the day they "suddenly" became ill. They wind up requiring more extreme measures because our health-care system does not offer anything like a one-hundred-thousand-mile tune-up. We just allow the vehicle (our bodies) to run down without doing anything about it.

If the body always functioned on its own without any need for inter-vention, why is there such a widespread reliance on medications and sur-geries? Their use disproves the contention that the body functions well on its own without any need for support. If the body supposedly never needs help, why do doctors so commonly prescribe drugs that intervene in the circulatory system (statins), neurological system (antidepressants), and metabolism (insulin)? Even though it's considered the norm for doc-tors to offer extreme and costly interventions, milder ones that support all these systems and prevent terrible ailments are ignored, or character-ized as beyond the pale.

And for some unknown reason, we especially neglect detoxification. The notion that out of all the bodily functions, the detox systems alone require no intervention or support is belied by the many illnesses to which toxicity is a prime contributor. Fortunately, you can increase your odds of avoiding problems that lead to intense interventions and medi-cations by supporting your body and detoxing regularly. The entire body benefits when you support detox. It is ironic, given the role detox plays in overall health, that it's the favorite target for conventional medical scorn.

I am thankful that through the Toxin Solution, you can benefit from time-tested and scientifically validated health wisdom that will help you navigate through our toxic world and maintain your health. Let's review where things stand now that we are midway through the program.

What Happens Next

Let me reiterate a point I covered in the previous chapter. Although detox is a safe and healthy process, to unleash your toxic load without preparation is counterproductive. And the best preparation is to get solid baseline nutrition, avoid letting new toxins in, and restore your gut health. Now that you are avoiding toxins, have built your baseline nutrition, used natural herbs to defeat harmful gut toxins, and restored the integrity of your gut, you are at last ready, in this chapter, to undertake my Two-Week Liver Detox Protocol.

A complex organ, the liver is absolutely key to successful detoxification. Your health and vitality are determined by your liver's capacity to detoxify the barrage of substances to which we all are exposed. In addition to processing, neutralizing, and excreting a host of chemical toxins from food, agriculture, industry, and consumer products, the liver also deals with toxic metabolic by-products that are generated by the body itself. In the prior two weeks, you considerably lightened that load, preparing your body to help your liver safely and completely release toxins.

Now that you have completed the Two-Week Jumpstart Diet (chapter 3), this is the right time to add healthy protein foods back in. Proteins are actually necessary for successful detoxification, since the key way the liver breaks down chemicals is through enzymes, which require protein for their production. Also, one of the key Phase II liver enzymes for finishing the chemical detoxification process requires the amino acids found in protein. This particular detoxification process, called acetylation, is especially important for women, because when it is not working properly, the risk of breast cancer increases a serious threefold.[1]

The research shows that effective liver detoxification affects virtually all aspects of health and disease risk. The protocols in this chapter feature all of the most essential foods that support the liver's detoxification enzymes and supply the key nutrient cofactors required for these critical enzymes to work.

If I were able to, I would personally monitor the progress of your detox, to ensure a good balance between how fast you release toxins from your cells, interstitial spaces, fat tissues, bones, and brain on the one hand, and how fast your liver breaks them apart and excretes them from your body on the other. But since I can't monitor you from afar,

I will provide all the tools you need to control the pace of your detox over the next two weeks.

Weeks 5 and 6: The Two-Week Liver Detox Protocol

In the Two-Week Liver Detox Protocol, you will:

- Restore your liver and repair any damage.
- Add nutritional and herbal support for your liver's special detox enzymes.
- Balance and support Phases I and II of your body's liver detox mechanisms.
- Rebuild your detox capacity.

Each day, you will take all the recommended nutritional supplements and herbs, plus two servings of the suggested foods, including specific vegetables and fruits.

The protocol itself is easy to follow, whether or not you fully understand the complex functions going on behind the scenes in your body. However, if you wish to know more, I will take you on a tour of how your liver works—and how you can optimize its processes. If you are the kind of person who likes to get the complete picture, you will find this fascinating. But if you don't need all the details, you can read selectively and simply follow the program to health.

In weeks 5 and 6, you will get ample quantities of leafy green vegetables to get folic acid—a crucial detox nutrient. Since protein-rich foods and choline are essential for liver detox and repair, you will eat eggs and lecithin. You will also eat foods rich in B vitamins (whole grains) and vitamin C (peppers, cabbage, citrus fruits), as well as specific dairy products, such as whey powder and Swiss cheese, and beans that are high in cysteine. Cysteine is critical for production of glutathione, the master detox molecule.

Table 5.1. **The Two-Week Liver Detox Protocol**

Weeks 5 and 6 Foods
• Two large whole eggs (the important liver detox nutrient choline is in the egg yolk, also high in cysteine) five times per week
• 1 cup of cooked beans or lentils four times per week (high in fiber to bind toxins, and in sulfur to support liver detoxification)
• 3 ounces of sardines, anchovies, or small mackerel four times per week
• Sunflower or sesame seeds (high in cysteine) sprinkled on all vegetables and salads
• One generous serving a day of cooked cabbage, broccoli, Brussels sprouts, asparagus, or other green leafy vegetables, seasoned with dill and caraway to activate their enzymes. (After you chop the vegetables, allow them to sit for five minutes before cooking. They are high in B vitamins required for liver detoxification and in glucosinolates, which promote liver-detoxification enzymes.)
• Artichokes: One every other day, steamed and eaten with lemon and organic olive oil, if possible. (On off days, see below for the correct dose for supplement form.)
• Greens: One generous handful per day of greens, such as Swiss chard, spinach, organic kale, bok choy, dandelion greens, or other greens suitable for light steaming that you can find. In addition or as a substitute, you can also eat red- and green-leaf lettuce, spinach, and other greens raw in salads, if you wish. (On off days, see below for the correct dose for supplement form.)
• Turmeric: Use freely in soups, stews, and curries (or take as the supplement curcumin).
• One organic apple five times per week (high in pectin to bind toxins)
• One serving every other day of avocado or walnuts (high in glutathione)
• One serving per day of a whole grain such as oats, oat bran, millet, or quinoa (high in fiber, trace minerals, and B vitamins)
• Two oranges or other citrus fruits, but not grapefruit, four times per week
• Cysteine-rich dairy foods, such as Swiss cheese, feta, or fat-free natural yogurt, 3 ounces three times per week
Weeks 5 and 6 Supplements
• Glutathione, topical or liposomal: 250 mg per day
• Vitamin B complex: 50 mg per day
• Vitamin C: 1,000 mg twice a day
• N-acetyl cysteine: 500 mg twice a day
• Indole-3-carbinol: 200 mg twice a day
• Artichoke extract: 500 mg twice a day
• Dandelion: 4 grams of dried root three times a day (can be taken in tea or capsule form)
• Curcumin (either Theracurmin or Meriva brand): 300 mg twice a day
• Fish oil: 1 gram twice a day
• Multivitamin: Take recommended dose on bottle.

What Will You Eat?

The following sample menu plans illustrate ways to include my recommendations into your daily diet.

Table 5.2. **Sample Menu Plans**

Day 1	
Breakfast	Scrambled eggs with refried black beans and sliced orange
Midmorning snack	Quinoa toast with sunflower butter and sliced apple
Lunch	Turkey chili with millet and steamed kale and apple-cabbage salad
Midafternoon snack	Steamed artichoke with orange-lemon dressing
Dinner	Hummus with sliced peppers; garlic-sesame broccoli with walnut sauce; green-leaf salad with scallion yogurt dressing
Day 2	
Breakfast	Oatmeal sprinkled with oat bran, cinnamon apple, chopped walnuts, and sunflower seeds
Midmorning snack	Sardines with lemon, with dilled cauliflower and quinoa toast
Lunch	Broccoli–Brussels sprouts stir-fry with sesame sauce and orange
Midafternoon snack	Artichoke with lemon hummus dip
Dinner	Black bean and red quinoa soup; steamed greens with orange butter; avocado salad

Understanding the Protocol: How the Liver Detoxes

Over the course of human evolution, the liver has evolved specific mechanisms that neutralize the waste products that result from the breaking down and filtering of toxins. But the modern explosion in industrial activity has caused the release of more toxins into our food and environment than our livers can cope with. Worse, these toxins were specifically designed to be difficult to break down by biological processes, making the liver's job even harder. Research links countless diseases to a poorly functioning liver. Examples include autoimmune disorders like lupus and rheumatoid arthritis, and degenerative neurological disorders such as Alzheimer's and Parkinson's disease.

The liver's detox systems also prevent cancer. When people are routinely exposed to large amounts and combinations of toxins and their livers are unable to detox them successfully, what happens? Their susceptibility to cancer increases. Up to 90 percent of all cancers are likely due to industrially produced carcinogens, such as those in cigarette smoke, or chemical pollutants in food, water, and air. Increasing toxic exposures contribute to disease incidence, but their effect also depends on how effectively your body responds. When researchers looked into an Italian chemical plant where workers had an unusually high rate of bladder cancer, they found that although all of the workers were exposed to the same level of carcinogens, those with the least effective detox systems were much more likely to develop cancer.[2]

What does this information reveal? And what can you do about it—in addition to lessening avoidable toxic exposures? Let me be frank: there are ways to measure innate detox capacity. But whatever the results, the bottom line remains the same: you have to undertake this type of program to correct your exposure to toxins. For example, suppose that your genetics ultimately reveal a lesser capacity for detox, or that you don't know your actual genetics. In either situation, you should limit your exposure to toxins: either your toxic load (the accumulated toxins you carry in your body) is high, or you have no clue about your actual toxic load and should take preventive measures just in case.

Because you live in our industrialized world, there is a very high likelihood that prior toxic exposures have already lessened your detox capacity, whether it was innately strong or weak. It's also quite likely that your toxic load is much higher than you realize. No matter what your detox capacity or toxic load, you will benefit from this program.

Yes, as I've mentioned earlier, some may have the time, money, and inclination to measure some of the above, but getting a complete picture isn't always easy. And in the end, given these realities, the majority of people will discover that the best thing they can possibly do for themselves is to follow the very recommendations I offer you here. The bottom line is that undertaking the liver cleanse I recommend in this chapter will always help, no matter what your individual situation is. Obviously, if you are currently suffering from a serious or life-threatening illness, you may want to pull out all of the stops to pin-point all of the contributing factors through genetic testing, laboratory tests, or other means.

People like to optimistically assume that their body can withstand the toxic barrage. But there is no reason why anyone should make that assumption. Yes, your body can heal, but only with your help. On average, if you suffer from mild complaints or seek to prevent more serious illness, you will find this liver cleanse highly effective in restoring diminished detox capacity.

I still vividly remember how in naturopathic medical school one of my most respected professors started class by asserting, "When in doubt, detoxify the liver." This seemed strange to me at the time, but almost a half century later, I've seen this old naturopathic adage proven in hundreds of patients. All the right foods and all the nutritional supplements in the world won't do much good if a person's enzyme systems are poisoned by chemical and metal toxins.

Students or practitioners of a healing art suppressed for so long by the medical-industrial complex tend to become unsure of themselves. When I started as a student, my profession was missing a generation. The AMA was so successful in dominating the health landscape that only six states still licensed NDs. There was only one school left in all of North America. To keep the school going, our teachers taught for free, and some even drove many hours to teach because they were sometimes the only person within hundreds of miles who understood some types of therapies. We students were grateful to these courageous practitioners for keeping the medicine alive, despite active persecution, but it was sometimes frustrating, since most of them could not easily explain the scientific rationale for why these therapies worked. With my very strong background in science and commitment to research, I was exceptionally skeptical at first. When my professor said we should start by detoxifying the liver, I asked to see the research. He simply asserted that clinically it almost always helps. Well, I was the student and he was the teacher, so I somewhat reluctantly followed his advice. (Now, decades later, the research has finally caught up with these insightful pioneers.)

Susan's Story

Susan was sixty-five years old, which at the time I thought was *really* old. She had heard about natural medicine but could not afford to see a regular naturopathic doctor, since naturopaths were not covered by her insurance. She came to our inexpensive teaching clinic after having undergone a checkup at a nearby welfare clinic. Not finding any overt disease, the doctors there told her that she was just getting old and should learn to live with feeling poorly. They offered to prescribe an antidepressant. That didn't sit well with her.

Susan was experiencing tiredness, bad breath, stomach upset, stiff joints in the morning, swollen ankles, dry skin, and progressive mental fogginess. I took a careful history, asked about her diet (which wasn't too bad), did a complete physical, ran the basic blood and urine tests—and found nothing wrong.

"When in doubt, detoxify the liver." With no good reason apart from wanting to follow my supervisor's advice, I put her on our standard liver-detoxification protocol (which I have since further evolved into the one I offer in this book). Of course, I also advised her to improve her diet, drink more water, and eat more fiber-rich foods, including more fruits and vegetables.

A month later she was dramatically better. I had no idea what toxins had overloaded her system or where they came from. All I did was help clear toxins out of her liver, improve her diet, and let her body do the rest. Four decades later, I have a much better understanding of toxins and where they come from and there are additional tools for getting rid of them. In retrospect, I now understand their source in Susan's case: as a part-time cleaning woman, she was regularly exposed to chemical toxins in the products she used. Eventually, they overloaded her liver's capacity to detoxify, and she started feeling old before her time. Fortunately, this basic liver cleanse, without even the benefit of the extra supplements you will take, worked to give Susan a new lease on life.

Before toxins enter the body from the digestive system, they have to pass through the liver. The portal vein that travels from the gut to the liver carries healthy vitamins and minerals, but it also carries the herbicides and pesticides that contaminate food, along with the BPA and phthalates absorbed from the plastic containers. A properly functioning liver gets rid of a high percentage of these toxins so they can't get into our body—but some still get in.

There are many things that harm the liver, which is why it's essential that you understand and limit damaging substances that undermine detox capacity. For example, alcoholics have increased disease due to alcohol-induced liver damage, which makes it harder to keep other toxins out. Even a small decrease in liver function allows a lot more toxins to pass into the blood. I think one reason practitioners of conventional medicine have not realized this problem is that it affects all aspects of health, not just one disease.

Fortunately, once you understand both what harms and what helps this key detox organ, you can correct past problems. Up to a certain point, it is possible to regenerate your liver. But you don't want to go for too long accruing damage and allowing the barrage of toxins to build up and weaken your liver beyond repair. That is why I consider the protocol I offer in this chapter to be a real life-changer. Follow it consistently during the current two weeks. And what should you do if you ever again experience health symptoms you don't know how to address? Detoxify the liver. It never hurts to start there.

Three Ways the Liver Detoxes

Let's look at the three key ways the liver works to rid your body of toxins:

1. Filtering the blood to remove large-molecule toxins

2. Synthesizing and secreting bile, to excrete fat-soluble toxins

3. Using enzymes to break down toxic chemicals

Filtering the Blood

Almost two quarts of blood pass from the gut through the liver every *minute*. When operating properly, this filtration system clears out bad bacteria, intact food and bacterial proteins, and other toxic substances that come from an overloaded gut.

But when the liver is damaged, this filtration system does not work as it should. For example, people with liver disease (such as chronic active hepatitis) can't eliminate toxins adequately. Instead, the liver allows them to pass into the bloodstream, where these toxins often damage tissues or provoke an immune response. And when the immune system's alarms are regularly set off, the result is constant inflammation, which disrupts normal metabolic processes and leads to, or aggravates, chronic disease.

Producing Bile

After filtering the blood, the liver produces bile, a dark-green or yellowish-brown liquid that solubilizes fats and fat-soluble toxins. In other words, bile makes these toxins liquid, which helps them exit your body. Stored in the gallbladder after it is produced by the liver, bile is secreted into the small intestine. As the toxins are dissolved, all that fiber you consume on this program absorbs the toxin-saturated bile. When your gut excretes that fiber (via your stools), your body can say good-bye to a portion of its toxic load.

That is why, in weeks 1 through 4 of the Toxin Solution, you began consuming more fiber—to absorb and carry off these toxins. You will continue eating extra fiber during weeks 5 and 6 to ensure that you excrete rather than reabsorb the chemical toxins the liver spent so much metabolic energy getting rid of. Remember, our liver-detoxification process evolved back when we were eating 100 to 150 grams of fiber a day, compared with the 15 to 20 we typically take in today. This low level of fiber sabotages our liver and makes us more toxic.

Using Enzymes to Break Down Toxic Chemicals

Liver enzymes break down unwanted chemicals so that they can be harmlessly released, or bound to molecules that render them inactive and easier to excrete. This process renders inactive:

- Industrial chemicals
- Agricultural chemicals
- Chemicals from consumer products
- Toxins from the gut
- Drugs
- Normal body chemicals, such as hormones estrogen and testosterone
- Inflammatory chemicals, such as histamines and prostaglandins

All of these chemicals, if allowed to build up, create a terrible toxic burden on your body.

Later in this chapter you will learn more about the science behind liver enzymes.

Julie's Story

Wearing a Seahawks sweatshirt, Julie—an overweight thirty-five-year-old woman—came to see me complaining of tiredness, bad breath, and depression. Although she'd tried to take off weight, she got so sick when she dieted that she couldn't continue. Year after year her weight relentlessly increased. Julie's diet was standard American fare—high in unhealthy fats and various forms of sugar, and grossly deficient in fruits and vegetables. She didn't take supplements, and she never exercised.

For her job as a machinist, Julie wore a uniform that she kept at work and rarely washed. Most nights, she met her friends after work and drank three or four beers. Remarkably, given her lifestyle and diet, her blood tests were normal, except for her liver enzymes, several of which were near the top of the normal range.

Julie's liver was overloaded. Her alcohol consumption had depleted her glutathione stores, undermining her liver's ability to protect her from solvent exposure at work. Her fat stores were so saturated with solvents from her work that when she dieted, the weight loss mobilized a flood of toxins stored in her fat cells. Her overloaded liver couldn't deal with the even higher load, so of course she felt terrible every time she tried to lose weight.

I first focused on stopping the influx of toxins while restoring her ability to detoxify. Weight loss was furthest from my mind; she had many more important issues to address. Improving ventilation, washing her uniform every day, being more conscious of when she was being exposed to chemicals, and taking steps to avoid them—these were obvious strategies, and Julie readily complied.

But dealing with her excessive alcohol consumption was trickier. I gave Julie two options: either drink nonalcoholic beer or take supplements to increase glutathione production. She chose the latter. She also increased her dietary fiber—starting at 3 grams twice a day and working up over two weeks to 5 grams three times a day. I also prescribed a good-quality multivitamin and mineral supplement and 500 mg of N-acetyl cysteine (NAC) twice a day.

When I saw Julie again two weeks later, she felt so much better I was able to convince her to try the alcohol-free beer, which I explained actually increases glutathione levels. Six months later, all her symptoms were gone.

Although weight loss was not our main goal, she also lost twenty pounds. Although the recent findings that chemical toxins act as "obesogens" was unknown back then, getting the chemicals out of her body allowed her excessive fat to melt away as Julie restored her health.

As by-products of its detox activities, the liver also produces inflammatory chemicals and free radicals. Unfortunately, if not immediately neutralized, these noxious substances can damage the liver itself. That's why this chapter features an antioxidant-rich diet. Along with protein, fruits and vegetables filled with antioxidants provide the nutrients your liver uses to mop up these nasty by-products and stay healthy.

Understanding Your Detox Experience

In a dynamic metabolic system like the human body, there is constant activity and many different parts that interact to make it all work. That is why it's especially important to pay attention to your body's messages during detox. Listening to your body will help you customize the program and make it work perfectly for you.

Many people believe that only a lab test reveals information, but that couldn't be further from the truth. There are a wealth of ways people can self-assess without lab tests. Back in the days when I first trained to be a naturopath, the few available lab tests were primitive compared with today's offerings. That was why, to figure out what was going on in the body, old-time clinicians mastered the art of reading their patients' signs and symptoms. Given that detoxification was foundational, these pioneers learned to determine when the detoxification process was in balance and when it was not. Fortunately, you can use their discoveries to promote your own health.

My teachers knew that when toxin release begins, the person's symptoms might actually get worse. The body likes to get rid of toxins, so when you open the tap for toxin release, the flood can become heavy. This has been labeled variously as the *healing crisis, detoxification reaction,* or *Herxheimer reaction.* Unless you have released large amounts of neurotoxins, these symptoms are nearly always minor and temporary. Yet detox reactions are a prime reason that some fear the process. Rest assured that although a few temporary uncomfortable sensations are extremely common, once you learn to self-assess, you will feel more confident about the process.

Once you learn to self-assess, you can also use my basic guidelines to help you manage the detox process. The first step is learning how to interpret your own bodily reactions. For example, one clear sign that your detox systems are on overwhelm is a decreased level of vitality. This is easy to gauge, because everyone knows when they feel debilitated and weak rather than energetic and healthy.

Note how you are feeling now. Then make sure to pay attention to how you feel day by day over the next two weeks. There are a number of ways to monitor how you are doing. For example, every day, you can take a symptom survey, such as the one I provide in appendix E. (This survey is also available on the website www.thetoxinsolution.com. It

Herbal Defenders

Dandelion. For centuries, herbalists revered dandelion as an invaluable liver remedy.[3] Studies in humans and laboratory animals reveal that dandelion enhances the flow of bile, lessening liver congestion and reducing bile-duct inflammation, hepatitis, gallstones, and jaundice.[4] Dandelion is so effective because it supports so many aspects of liver detox.

You can take a dandelion supplement (as in the protocol). Or you can eat dandelion leaves either steamed or in salads. If you want to harvest dandelion leaves yourself, be sure to not use those from lawns that have been sprayed with toxins.

Artichoke. Artichoke-leaf extract (as recommended in the protocol) also increases the excretion of bile from the liver. Research demonstrates that there is significantly more bile excretion for two to three hours after taking it[5]—one reason that artichoke extract is now used to lower cholesterol, which is eliminated through the bile. You can also eat one artichoke per day as shown in the sample menu plan. Artichokes are best if cooked and eaten with oil, since this will increase absorption of the important constituents.

Turmeric. Finally, freely use the common spice turmeric. (Or take it as a supplement as shown in the protocol.) Turmeric contains the yellow pigment curcumin, which also increases the flow of bile from the liver and decreases blood cholesterol levels.[6]

Using dandelion, artichoke, and turmeric for the next two weeks will both lighten your toxic load and heal your liver.

automatically calculates your daily health score and graphically tracks your health over time.) While daily may be too often for you, please be sure to do this at least weekly. People are often so concerned with their current symptoms that they forget how much they have improved over time. If you don't have time to fill in the form, you can simply ask yourself these three questions when you awaken in the morning:

1. Do I have a headache?

2. Does my breath smell bad?

3. Do I feel tired upon rising in the morning and unenthusiastic the rest of the day?

If you feel there are other measures of your health that you want to add, feel free to do so. You are likely reading this book because you don't feel as healthy as you want to feel. The critical factor is consistently checking in with yourself. Each of us knows best how we feel.

What Happens During Detox

Let's take a closer look at how the body works. As you have learned in this chapter, liver enzymes neutralize specific toxins. Many of these enzymes, key players in the body's cleanup crew, are what is called *inducible*. That means the body won't generate these enzymes until they are needed. Typically, once toxins persist at elevated levels for more than a day or so, the genes that produce these enzymes switch on to detoxify them. That is why many people report feeling more toxic the first few days after beginning active detox. What's really going on? You actually do feel worse *before these enzymes kick in*. But by the end of the first week, *after they kick in,* you should start feeling progressively better.

What are the signs that you are detoxifying successfully? You may experience:

- Skin rashes

- Increased mucus excretion (stuffed or runny nose)

- Bad breath

- Smellier stools or urine

- Headache

- Heavy, achy lungs

These symptoms indicate that your body is releasing unwanted substances through every route available. These symptoms will improve (or clear up entirely) by the beginning of the second week. It bears repeating so you are clear on what to expect: the more toxins you have to excrete, the more symptoms you will likely experience, and the longer it will take to get the toxins out of your body.

By understanding the process, it's easier to handle the symptoms. They are soon over in any case, and the payoff is well worth the minor discomfort. If things get too uncomfortable, you can manage your own rate of detox. I'll show you how to do that now.

You Can Always Adjust the Rate of Detox

Perhaps you recall Conrad, whom I mentioned in chapter 4. He experienced detox reactions because he went back to his previous bad habits during the program, and his body simply could not handle it. I mention this to point out that, whatever happens, there is a way to handle it. With Conrad, I slowed his detox, and he recovered and resumed his protocol.

Let's look at the worst possible scenario, although it rarely happens. If toxins are being released too quickly, you will feel sicker and your vitality will be lower. Although this is very unlikely, if you have especially high levels of specific toxins, a too-rapid release can even be dangerous. Indications you are detoxifying too rapidly include:

- Brain fog
- Debility
- Depression
- Disorientation
- Dizziness
- Fast heart rate
- Headache

- Insomnia
- Irregular heartbeat
- Irritability
- Muscle spasms
- Nausea
- Shortness of breath
- Weakness

If you experience any of these symptoms, one of the best and simplest ways to decrease your symptoms without slowing down your detox is to cut dose of herbs in half, consume more berries, and eat more fiber. Just add to the protocol 5 grams of a fiber supplement with a full glass of water three times every day. This will help to absorb all those toxins being dumped by your liver and excrete them from your body via the stools. In this way, toxins do not end up being reabsorbed. The best forms of fiber are oat bran, flaxseed powder, and a supplement called PGX, which I mentioned in chapter 3. I don't recommend wheat fiber, since so many people react to wheat.

I hope these tips give you confidence that you can safely detox at a level that feels comfortable for you.

The Science Behind Liver Enzymes

There are two phases to the liver's enzymatic process, Phase I and Phase II. The program of foods and supplements I offer gives you all of the essential foods and key nutritional supplements to support both phases.

The interaction between Phase I and Phase II is quite complex. As you can see, all toxins enter the liver, which breaks them down in these two distinct phases, each of which requires its own specific nutrients. The protocol provides the supports necessary for each phase of liver enzyme activity.

Figure 5.1. **Liver detoxification pathways**

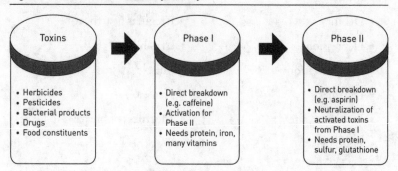

I don't expect you to fully grasp every detail, but the bottom line is that many interlocking biochemical pathways must work together for optimal detoxification. As a scientist, I find it exciting to glimpse how nature works within us. Unfortunately, though, since conventional doctors don't understand how to support detoxification, I've often heard them say that detoxification happens naturally, without the need for any additional support. Once again, it's easier to dismiss the problem of an overloaded and weakened detox capacity than it is to find ways to help this complex system operate optimally. This is a powerful example of how the disease-treatment orientation of conventional medicine—which works so well for acute problems like infections and injury, where there is a direct correlation between a single cause and a single result—fails us for everyday health. Most toxins indiscriminately cause damage throughout the body. This absence of a direct link between a given toxin and a specific disease does not fit the dominant medical model, resulting in conventional medicine being oblivious to the real reasons our population suffers so much ill health and disease. The work you are doing to detoxify your body will not only help you feel better today but also dramatically decrease your risk of developing disease in the future.

Anyone who begins to get a picture of how all the detox organs and systems work together will see why, as naturopathic medicine has long held, supporting detox is the frontline defense for the body.

Phase I Detoxification

Organs and systems aren't static entities. They interact through what scientists call *metabolic processes*. The thyroid produces the hormone thyroxin, which tells each cell how much energy to produce, and the pancreas produces insulin to tell the cells how much sugar to absorb. These are just a few examples of the approximately five thousand metabolic processes that are going on in the body in each moment. Let's look at a few performed by the liver.

In Phase I, there are three ways that these liver enzymes metabolize—that is, break down—and get rid of a toxin:

1. By neutralizing it, i.e., chemically breaking it apart

2. By converting it into a form that is water-soluble (through a process known as *solubilizing*) for excretion by the kidneys

3. By converting it to a more chemically active form, called an *active intermediate*

These active intermediates are then worked on further and then neutralized by Phase II.

Three Methods of Phase I Detox

As I mentioned earlier, as an organ, the liver itself filters out toxins in several ways. But during the Phase I process, certain enzymes perform very specific detox and conversion activities. Let's look at these three methods.

1. **Neutralizing Toxins.** Many toxic chemicals are totally broken down by these important first-line defense enzymes in the liver. However, in the process, your liver cells can be harmed. Every time Phase I enzymes transform a toxin, those same enzymes generate free radicals, which must be neutralized immediately or else they will damage the liver.

Suppose someone eats a poisonous mushroom. As the liver works overtime to neutralize the toxins from the mushroom, it generates a cascade of free radicals that use up its storehouse of protective antioxidants, especially glutathione. If there is insufficient glutathione, the resulting damage can be so extensive that the liver is destroyed. This is why people can die from eating poisonous mushrooms—they cause liver failure. Maintaining adequate levels of antioxidants will protect your hard-working liver. And that's why, over the next two weeks, you will boost your antioxidant levels.

Eating cysteine-rich foods and supplementing with NAC helps reduce high levels of toxins, carcinogens, and oxidants. The maintenance and antioxidant dose ranges from 100 to 500 mg per day for antioxidant support.[7] To promote detoxification, take higher amounts: 500 mg twice a day.[8]

2. **Solubilizing Toxins.** Fat-soluble toxins, such as the herbicides and pesticides I discussed in chapter 3, tend to stick around in your cells and fatty tissues. Studies reveal that they have long half-lives in the body. Once they get in, it's hard to get them out. To deal with them, the liver uses enzymes that make them water-soluble. Then, the modified toxin can be carried out of the liver and excreted in the bile or else carried in the blood to the kidneys for excretion in the urine.[9]

3. **Converting Toxins.** If your Phase I liver enzymes can't either neutralize a toxin or make it water-soluble, they do the next best thing: they

Glutathione

As I've mentioned earlier in this book, the most important antioxidant in your entire body is glutathione (GSH). Glutathione neutralizes free radicals, especially those produced by Phase I. But it also supports Phase II processes that detoxify persistent organic pollutants (POPs). If your glutathione gets used up, your liver is more susceptible to free-radical damage. As a result, the Phase II enzymes that depend upon glutathione can't so easily rid your body of the herbicides and pesticides used in modern agriculture.

You can obtain glutathione either through your diet (technically from the cysteine in the dietary glutathione) or through internal synthesis—

which means the body itself can assemble glutathione from various other chemicals. Whether its key precursors are obtained through foods (such as fresh fruits and vegetables like avocado, cooked fish, dairy products, walnuts, and meat) or taken as a supplement, you must get adequate glutathione. Oral glutathione supplements aren't very effective, because GSH breaks down in the intestines. Please take topical or liposomal forms of glutathione, which are available at good-quality health-food stores.

The body can also synthesize glutathione—which is by far the primary way we get this needed molecule. Some substances, such as N-acetyl cysteine (NAC), provide high levels of cysteine for the body. Longevity increases in animals fed NAC, since it increases glutathione synthesis. Your body more rapidly produces glutathione when you have sufficient cysteine. The bottom line is that NAC raises blood, liver, cellular, and mitochondrial levels of this important antioxidant. NAC has also been shown to help decrease the toxicity of chemotherapeutic drugs used to treat cancer, as well as that of antibiotics used for infections.[10]

Fresh fruits and vegetables contain 25 to 750 mg of glutathione per pound. Higher quantities are found in sesame and sunflower seeds. That is why during weeks 5 and 6 of the program, you will consume more of these foods. Commercially prepared foods, dairy products (milk has little, but whey extract is high), most cereals, legumes, and nuts (apart from walnuts) have little glutathione. Among processed foods, frozen foods generally retain their glutathione content. (Technically minded readers might be interested to know that almost all the glutathione in food is broken down to cysteine, which the body absorbs to produce glutathione.)

People with certain conditions have been found to have a deficiency of glutathione, probably due to their greatly increased need for it, both as an antioxidant and for detoxification.[11] These conditions include:

- Adult respiratory distress syndrome
- Age-related hearing loss
- Atherosclerosis

- Brain dysfunction
- Cancer
- Cardiovascular disease
- Cataract formation
- Chronic obstructive pulmonary disease (COPD)
- Cystic fibrosis
- Drug sensitivity
- Dubin–Johnson syndrome
- Emphysema
- Hemolytic anemia
- Hepatic cirrhosis
- HIV infection
- Hypoglycemia
- Idiopathic pulmonary fibrosis
- Kidney stones
- Metabolic acidosis
- Multidrug resistance
- Myocardial infarction
- Neurological symptoms
- Osteoporosis
- Reduced inflammatory response
- Schizophrenia

Studies show that large segments of the elderly population have low glutathione levels.[12] A deficiency of vitamin B$_6$ also results in decreased production of glutathione.

modify it and pass the job off to Phase II. But all too often the modified versions hang around and create even more damage.

Let's look at one example: Everyone knows that smoking causes cancer. But have you ever wondered how? It happens when your liver can't complete the job of modifying specific toxins at Phase I and passes the incompletely modified—and even more dangerous—form of the compound along to Phase II.

Let's look at the specific compounds that make cigarette smoke so toxic—and why they are a challenge to detoxify.

A chemical group called polycyclic aromatic hydrocarbons are the culprits. According to the Agency for Toxic Substances and Disease Registry (ATSDR), polycyclic aromatic hydrocarbons (PAHs) are carcinogens found in coal tar, crude oil, and many other substances.[13]

PAHs form when coal, oil, gas, charbroiled meat, and—yes—cigarettes are burned. If you live near a coal plant, charbroil your meat, use an oil heater, or smoke a cigarette, you will absorb PAHs. PAHs damage DNA—which can promote the development of cancer, pulmonary disease, reproductive disorders, and developmental problems.[14]

Now, pay close attention to what happens when your hard-working liver attempts to detoxify PAHs. (This also applies to other toxins in Phase I.) If your liver can't complete the task, you are much worse off. PAHs (and certain other toxic chemicals) are more carcinogenic *after* Phase I activation. Why does this matter?

Some people with a very active Phase I have a slow Phase II—a combination doctors call *pathological detoxification*. In this scenario, Phase I builds up toxic versions of a dangerous compound faster than Phase II can disarm them. The end result is more severe toxic reactions to chemical and industrial poisons.

To avoid creating this type of imbalance, my protocol supports *both* Phase I and Phase II. Certain nutrients like those found in berries, and herbs like turmeric, can also help directly neutralize these modified toxins so they can't harm you while they are stuck in your system, waiting for Phase II to disarm them.

Phase I Detox Activators

As you can see in the table on page 162, the foods that are already featured in this phase of the program act in combination to enhance liver enzyme function.

Table 5.3. **Substances That Activate Phase I Detoxification**

Foods	Cabbage, broccoli, and Brussels sprouts
	High-protein diet
	Oranges and tangerines; citrus peel (but not grapefruit peel)
Nutrients	Iron
	Niacin, Vitamin B_1 (thiamine), and B_2 (riboflavin)
	Vitamin C
	Cysteine, methionine, taurine—found primarily in animal products like fish, eggs, and most dairy products; and for vegetarians, seaweed, krill, and brewer's yeast
Herbs	Caraway and dill seeds (oil also works)

Brassicas

In all phases of the Toxin Solution, you eat a lot more vegetables from the brassica family (cabbage, broccoli, and Brussels sprouts). You will continue to eat them during weeks 5 and 6 because they contain nutrients and chemical constituents that stimulate both Phase I and Phase II detoxification enzymes. Two of these compounds, vitamin C and a chemical called indole-3-carbinol, stimulate detoxifying enzymes in the gut as well as the liver,[15] protecting you from several toxins, including carcinogens. Eating brassicas protects against cancer, especially breast cancer.

Limonenes

Oranges and tangerines (as well as the seeds of caraway and dill) contain limonene, a phytochemical that has been found to prevent and treat cancer in animals. Limonene induces the Phase I and Phase II enzymes that can neutralize carcinogens.[16] As someone who serves on the science boards of two foundations that fund cancer research, I would like to see follow-up studies on limonenes done with humans.

What Stalls Phase I Detoxification

Just as certain foods and herbs support Phase I enzyme activity, some things work against it. For example, grapefruit *decreases* a specific Phase I enzyme activity that helps to prevent breast cancer and detoxify caffeine. Other common inhibitors of Phase I detoxification are listed in table 5.4. You would do well to avoid them if possible during this program in order to avoid sending your body mixed messages as you detox.

As part of the protocol, you will eat the Indian spice turmeric or supplement with its active ingredient, curcumin. Yes, you may have noticed that curcumin decreases activity of some Phase I enzymes. However, its net effect is very positive: curcumin increases the flow of bile, inhibits Phase I carcinogen activation, stimulates Phase II, and directly inhibits the growth of cancer cells.[17]

Curcumin is not the sole nutrient that's beneficial in both phases. In fact, Phase I and Phase II processes overlap and detoxify some of the same chemicals. This overlap helps the liver remove the most deadly toxins. Not all of these detox pathways are equally efficient, but since any single system can be overwhelmed or working poorly due, for example, to genetics, this backup system does help increase protection from toxins.

Table 5.4. **Inhibitors of Phase I Detoxification**

Drugs	Benzodiazepine antidepressants (for example, Centrax, Librium, Prozac, and Valium)
	Antihistamines (used for allergies)
	Cimetidine and other stomach-acid-secretion-blocking drugs (used for stomach ulcers)
	Ketoconazole
	Sulfaphenazole
Foods	Naringenin from grapefruit juice
	Curcumin from the spice turmeric (decreases some Phase I activity, but its other benefits make up for it, especially in protection from oxidative damage)
	Capsaicin from red chili pepper
	Eugenol from clove oil
Other	Aging
	Toxins from inappropriate bacteria in the intestines

What Happens to Your Detox Capacity When You Age?

As DNA ages and becomes damaged by toxins, the typical person pro-gressively loses her or his ability to increase production of enzymes on demand. All the detoxification enzymes become progressively less effective—which is why you need to get toxins out as soon as possible!

To sum up, to ensure that Phase I works well:

- Eat plenty of brassica-family foods (cabbage, broccoli, and Brussels sprouts).
- Eat foods rich in B vitamins (nutritional yeast, whole grains) and vitamin C (peppers, cabbage, tomatoes, and citrus fruit, such as oranges and tangerines, but not grapefruit).

Phase II Detoxification

As discussed above, when Phase I enzymes are unable to complete detoxification, they pass a modified version of the original toxin along to Phase II. This modified toxin is called an *activated intermediate*. Activated intermediates can also build up when Phase II slows down. This slowdown can be caused by the following:

- Depleted glutathione stores (due to toxin overload, alcohol consumption, or the regular use of acetaminophen)
- Poorly functioning mitochondria
- Specific nutrient deficiencies
- Inadequate exercise
- Low levels of thyroid hormone

Now you can see why glutathione is so key to this protocol. By supple-menting with GSH and eating glutathione-rich foods as recommended, you activate key Phase II enzymes.

And what about exercise? It's a vicious cycle when toxicity itself reduces your ability to exercise, which then further undermines your detox capacity. The good news is that on my plan, you will have a renewed ability to take in and absorb the right nutrients. The net result will be that on this program you upgrade your detox capacity. Restoring your energy and well-being will make it easier to exercise. Even if you are feeling too tired to exercise, at least go for a 20-minute walk. This increases blood flow through your liver to help with the detoxification process.

Following a comprehensive plan like the one offered in this chapter offers a unique opportunity to repair the detox mechanisms and to detoxify. That is why I recommend following every aspect of the Nine-Week Program.

Support for Phase II Detoxification

Here are some of the key nutrients you will use in the protocol to support Phase II detox:

- Brassica-family foods (cabbage, broccoli, and Brussels sprouts), limonene-containing foods (citrus peel, dill oil, and caraway oil)
- Glycine (found in turkey, seaweed, and soy)
- Protein-rich foods (such as small fish, eggs, and dairy products like Swiss cheese and feta)
- Choline-rich foods (lecithin, eggs), folic acid (green leafy vegetables), and vitamin B_{12} (animal products or supplements)
- NAC and foods high in cysteine (dairy products, beans, whole grains)
- B vitamins (yeast, whole grains)
- Vitamin C (peppers, cabbage, citrus fruits)
- Fish oil

What Stalls Phase II Detoxification

Earlier in this chapter, I mentioned why those who already suffer from health concerns—as well as health mavens—might wish to go a step further to increase the program's results.

Here's your chance. As important as it is to support healthy detox function through the protocol, unfortunately you can't assume that you begin that process with a solid nutritional baseline. Although the Two-Week Jumpstart Diet is designed to correct the most common nutritional deficiencies, due to poor diet, many people in the United States have a much wider range of nutrient depletions. The lack of certain key substances will limit your body's ability to successfully perform Phase II detox. Following is a list of certain key factors that undermine a successful Phase II process. Nutritional deficiencies top the list. That is why I also offer dosage recommendations for correcting them. Adding these additional supplements is an optional feature of this program; and it can be very helpful to do so to make sure you have all you need for a successful Phase II.

- Selenium deficiency: Take a selenium dose of 150 micrograms (µg) per day

- Glutathione deficiency: Take NAC at a recommended dose of 500 milligrams (mg) two times per day

- Zinc deficiency: Take a zinc dose of 25 mg per day

- Low-protein diet: Increase protein by eating healthy proteins such as small fish, eggs from free-range chickens, and organically grown soy

- Folic acid deficiency: Take activated folates (MTHF and, if available, BH4) at a dose of 400 µg per day

- Vitamin B_{12} deficiency: Take a vitamin B_{12} dose of 500 µg methylcobalamin per day

- Vitamin B_2, B_5, or C deficiency: Take a vitamin B_2 dose of 10 mg per day, a vitamin B_5 dose of 250 mg per day, and a vitamin C dose of 1,000 mg two times per day

- Molybdenum deficiency: Take a molybdenum dose of 200 μg per day

How Do You Know If Your Liver Is Not Detoxing Effectively?

Generally, sophisticated blood tests are needed to prove that a specific liver detox system is dysfunctional. But there are several signs and symptoms that indicate detox incapacity. Anytime you have a bad reaction to a drug or toxin, you can be pretty sure there is a detoxification problem. Some symptoms of liver detox dysfunction include the following:

- Adverse reactions to sulfite food additives (as in commercial potato salad, salad bars, wine, and dried fruit)

- Asthma reactions after eating at a restaurant

- Caffeine intolerance (even small amounts keep you awake at night)

- A strong urine odor after eating asparagus

- Feeling sick after eating garlic

- Yellow discoloration of eyes and skin, not due to hepatitis

- Intolerance to perfumes or strong odors

Genetic Variability

For some people, eating asparagus reveals a genetic variability in liver detoxification. Asparagus is the only food with a sulfur-containing compound called asparagusic acid. One specific liver enzyme (sulfox-idase) determines if, and even how, a person breaks down asparagusic acid. Genetics also determines whether or not your body will produce an odiferous compound in the urine after you eat asparagus. This odor is unusual among Chinese people, while a predominant number of French Caucasians experience such an odor. (About 50 percent of adults in the United States notice this effect.)[18] Further complicating the story is that there is also genetic variation in how well people are able to perceive the asparagus urine odor!

Differences in genetics underlie more-critical health responses as well. Why can some people smoke for a whole lifetime with seeming impunity, while others develop lung cancer from just living with a smoker? In fact, researchers found that the two critical factors in cancer development are:

1. Exposure to multiple carcinogens
2. Poorly functioning detoxification enzymes[19]

Here's another example of how genetic variations in detox capacity influence health outcomes. Nearly 5 percent of all hospital admissions are due to adverse drug reactions (ADRs). And for those over the age of sixty-five, the numbers are even worse, accounting for one out of six hospital admissions![20] This is a medical-industry blind spot. Few peo-ple realize that, according to standardized treatment criteria, properly prescribed drugs are actually the fourth leading cause of death in the United States.[21] Why? Because of the way drugs are tested and pre-scribed. Even when a medication has been shown to address a specific symptom in a statistically significant number of patients tested, that does not mean that the drug is healthy for any or all of these patients. Nor do such studies predict for whom the drug may cause a harmful reaction. There is a thousandfold variation in how well people's Phase I enzymes work and a tenfold variation in Phase II enzymes. This means the standard dose of a drug will cause toxicity in typically 10 percent of people. And this works the other way around as well, meaning that some drugs don't work because they are being detoxified too quickly.

Some—but not all—people suffer from the side effects of prescription drugs. Until recently it was impossible to predict *who* is at risk for side effects, but liver enzymes may provide a clue. In observing the differing ways people react to prescription drugs, we can actually see liver enzymes at work. Genetic variations dictate how the enzymes perform from person to person. But most doctors aren't paying attention to these significant distinctions to help people make the right health-care choices.

People react to drugs differently because they have differing capacities to detoxify the substances the drugs contain. You are more likely to suffer one or more of a drug's side effects, even a serious one, if you have a weakened detox capacity. In other words, with a limited detox capacity, you are at higher risk when taking a drug. In my view, no doctor should prescribe a potentially toxic drug without knowing how well a person's drug-detoxifying enzymes are working. Unfortunately, most doctors (apart from those who practice as I do) are unaware of this. I often tell people that if they want to improve their health, they need to become their own best doctors. You can better determine which drugs are right or wrong for you by doing the genetic testing I recommend in appendix G.

How Well Can We Clear Toxins?

Here's another example of the role Phase I and Phase II liver enzymes play in detox. When taking drugs like acetaminophen (the active ingredient in Tylenol),[22] people usually think only about what the drug does, not what the body has to do to get rid of it afterward. So what does your body have to do if you take Tylenol? Acetaminophen can be detoxified in four ways:

1. Excretion by the kidneys into the urine unchanged
2. Binding to glucuronic acid (made from blood sugar) in Phase II and excretion in the urine

3. Binding to sulfur and excretion in the urine

4. Metabolizing in Phase I into the highly toxic NAPQI (N-acetyl-p-benzoquinone imine), which, optimally, is immediately bound to glutathione and excreted in the urine. (Most of it is handled that way.)

However, if Phase II processing doesn't work very well or excessive alcohol consumption has depleted the glutathione stores, it's harder to get rid of the NAPQI. It then damages and even kills liver cells. This is one reason why acetaminophen toxicity results in so many emergency-room visits: over fifty-six thousand people every year end up in the emergency room from acetaminophen reactions. Interestingly, the standard of care for treatment of this is IV-administered N-acetyl cysteine (NAC), which greatly increases glutathione production in the liver to get rid of the NAPQI as quickly as possible. Acetaminophen toxicity is also one of the primary causes of acute liver failure. This also reveals why a high toxic load is so risky. The more toxins you absorb, the more you deplete glutathione stores and the more damaging *all* toxins become.

How do you protect yourself if you take acetaminophen? Take NAC. This great nutrient increases your liver production of glutathione. Obviously I don't recommend that you overdose with acetaminophen or consume excessive alcohol. But understanding how the liver works can help you support its detox capacity.

Extra Supports for Weak Liver Detox Capacity

Many people have poor detoxification function for all the reasons I've covered in this chapter. If following the suggestions I've offered in this chapter does not help, make sure to do the following:

1. Go back and make sure to correct all possible nutritional deficiencies, using the dosage recommendations in the "What Stalls Phase II Detoxification" section of this chapter.

Figure 5.2. **Detoxification of acetaminophen**

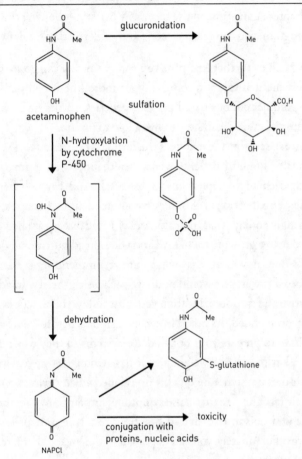

2. Look into changing any prescription drugs to ones that cause less damage to detoxification systems.

3. Revisit the "Toxin Troubleshooter" section in chapter 2, and check to see if there are any additional toxic sources you can eliminate.

4. Continue with the toxin-elimination plan that I recommend in chapter 2. Make sure you follow it for the full nine weeks of this program.

5. Feel free to revisit the Two-Week Liver Detox Protocol in this chapter at any time in the future. When not following this program, you can take turmeric and milk thistle on a daily basis.

If you wish to further fine-tune your program, you can go to my website (www.thetoxinsolution.com) and get more fine-tuned daily nutritional recommendations based on your genetics. In the final chapter, I will discuss in more detail how to live a low-toxin life.

As you can see from the many case histories I have presented, I've helped thousands of grateful patients whose health improved dramatically—many experiencing complete disease reversal. And I myself have used the same detoxification techniques recommended in this book. I can't state strongly enough that ill health and chronic disease are now almost entirely due to a growing toxin load and widespread nutritional deficiencies. This does not mean that what I am recommending is simple and easy to do; if it were, we would not have such a sick society. In addition, for effective and safe detoxification you must follow these steps exactly as I have recommended. As noted in earlier chapters, before we release toxins, we have to prepare your body's detox systems so they won't be overloaded. A key reason overweight people have trouble losing real weight is that their detox systems are quickly overloaded when toxins are released from their fat. These toxins cause symptoms similar to having the flu all the time and poison the thyroid function, resulting in depression and low energy. Fortunately, you can detox safely and escape that fate.

Upon completing weeks 5 and 6 of the program, you have brought Phase I and Phase II into balance and strengthened and supported the liver-detoxification pathways. Next, in weeks 7 and 8, you will support the body's third major detox organ—the kidneys.

The good news is that by following my nine-week plan, you will detoxify without feeling toxic, and the many health benefits are a wonderful reward for all your effort.

6

Revive Your Kidneys

Before beginning the program outlined in these pages, you learned to recognize where toxins come from and how to decrease your exposure to them. Then, in the first two weeks of the Toxin Solution, you began to eat a toxin-free diet. Most people who are aware of natural health options have probably already heard of liver and kidney cleanses. But those practices are usually offered as separate recipes without a core understanding of their interconnectivity within the body.

What is interconnectivity? The body's organs of detoxification aren't merely isolated organs. They are systems that function collaboratively. As mentioned in chapter 4, a toxic gut hurts detox in two ways: it fails to prevent absorption of harmful toxins coming from the wrong gut bacteria, contaminated food, consumer products, and industrial emissions; and it generates harmful products called endotoxins. And when these toxins and endotoxins back up into your other detox organs, they add to your toxic burden and reduce your detox capacity. That is why, in the second two weeks, in order to stop putting such a heavy load on your liver, you followed the plan to detoxify your gut. The next step was to improve the performance of Phase I and Phase II liver activity.

At this juncture, you should be experiencing an upsurge of energy.

Now, in weeks 7 and 8, you will detox the third major detox organ in your body, your kidneys. Although you probably don't think much about your kidneys, the truth is that if your kidneys don't function well, you cannot successfully detoxify. According to the Mayo Clinic, these symptoms are typical of kidney disease—though they usually appear only after kidney damage is pretty significant:

- Nausea

- Vomiting

- Loss of appetite

- Fatigue and weakness

- Sleep problems

- Changes in urine output

- Decreased mental sharpness

- Muscle twitches and cramps

- Hiccups

- Swelling of feet and ankles

- Persistent itching

- Chest pain, if fluid builds up around the lining of the heart

- Shortness of breath, if fluid builds up in the lungs

- High blood pressure (hypertension) that's difficult to control

Why do the kidneys work so hard? Because they have to deal with heavy metals, chemical toxins, and hazardous industrial emissions, as I've discussed in chapters 1 and 2—and some of these simply can't be avoided.

Many kinds of outside chemical toxins in agriculture and industry specifically target the kidneys, such as:[1]

- Persistent organic pollutants (POPs)

- Chemicals used in the production of plastics, like dichloroethene

- Pesticide products and pesticide residues like dioxanes, dibromoethane, chlordecone, chlorobenzene, and hexachlorocyclopentadiene (HCCPD)

- Antimicrobial products like ethylene oxide

- Solvents like chloroform, bromoform, hexachlorobutadiene, and xylenes

- Coal tar derivatives like benzofuran

- Flame retardants like bromodichloromethane, and phosphate ester flame retardants

- Chemicals we may be exposed to regularly, like antifreeze (ethylene glycol), gasoline (methyl tert-butyl ether, or MTBE) and petroleum hydrocarbons, and the perfluoroalkyls used on nonstick pans, breathable fabrics, and fabrics to make them resistant to grease, oil, and water

- Charbroiled foods containing kidney-damaging chemicals like nitrosodiphenylamine

- Food additives like propylene glycol

I'm here to tell you that poor kidney function can be reversed. Over the long years of my practice, I've helped many people to restore kidney function and improve their detox capacity. The research and my clinical experience confirm that, with the right supports, you can safely and effectively get toxins out of your body, decrease symptoms, lower disease risk, and improve your health.

Why do I emphasize the kidneys? The kidneys filter the blood and are the second-most-important organs of toxin elimination. Over 20 percent of all the blood flow passes through them daily, showing yet again that detoxification is a crucial part of the human physiological design.

As your blood circulates through your kidneys, this bean-shaped pair of organs work day and night, twenty-four seven, to filter out the toxins in your food and drink. When the toxic load gets too much for them to handle, they slow down. And when overwhelmed, the kidneys themselves become toxic, producing kidney stones, infections, cysts, and tumors. Finally, they may shut down altogether, which is a life-threatening condition.

Unfortunately, we are now exposed to such a high toxic load that the average person's kidneys wear out before their time. This means a dramatic decrease in our ability to get rid of many toxins and helps explain why almost everyone gets sicker as the years pass. The average load most people put on their kidneys is so heavy that by the time of death, most people have lost 50 percent of their kidney function.

And that's not all. The kidneys also must rid your body of toxic residues from various bodily processes. Although the kidneys are usually able to remove most toxins from the blood, often they aren't able to accomplish the next stage of the process: moving those toxins into the urine, and from there out of the body. And when the detox process is interrupted, toxins accumulate in the kidneys themselves. As the toxic concentration mounts, that toxic brew can seriously damage the kidneys.

What Causes Loss of Kidney Function?

There is no single way that people damage their kidneys. Rather, the cumulative effect of many factors causes loss of kidney function. Unless these hard-working organs perform at maximum efficiency, toxins will continue to accumulate in your body with every passing day.

That is why in the Two-Week Kidney Detox Protocol (page 177), you will be doing two things:

1. Providing the kidneys with the right nutrients so they can do their job

2. Limiting your consumption of substances that damage the
   kidneys

Both are equally important. Because pharmaceutical medicine prom-
ises us that a pill can correct any problem, most people are unaccustomed
to eating the right foods and taking the right nutritional substances,
which I encourage throughout the Toxin Solution. But even if you are
following the program, you undermine your efforts when you continue
with habits that harm the very organ you are trying to restore. That is
why it's essential that you both do the right things and not do the wrong
ones.

The Two-Week Kidney Detox Protocol

Here is the overview of what you will do and not do in weeks 7 and 8.
After I describe the protocol, I explain each feature and why it's essential. I will also show you how to customize the protocol to ensure the
optimal rate of toxin breakdown and excretion. Note that while this
program calls for no animal protein, you may, if you wish, include some
animal products the first week. However, there are two good reasons to
omit them. The first is to decrease your protein consumption, since their
breakdown products put a higher load on the kidneys. Second, since
chemical and metal toxins concentrate in conventionally raised animals,
avoiding these foods further decreases your toxic load.

Understanding the Protocol: Detoxing Your Kidneys

This small pair of organs filters all your blood a remarkable sixty times
per day—one of the most constant and crucial of your body's detox
mechanisms. When your body performs many of its internal biochemical processes, certain chemicals are generated. In and of themselves,
these by-products are toxic and are meant to be released from your body.

Often that task falls to the kidneys, which must get rid of the following:

- Ammonia

- Urea

- Uric acid

- Creatinine

- Hormone metabolites

- Post–Phase II water-soluble toxins

- Heavy metals and other industrial toxins

- New-to-nature molecules (for example, POPs)

- Excess vitamins, salt, and phosphates

Have you ever noticed that your urine turns bright yellow/orange after you take B vitamins or a multivitamin? That is your kidneys getting rid of the extra vitamin B_2.

Although the kidneys regularly remove toxins from the blood, they sometimes have a problem passing those same toxins into the urine. As a result, the toxins accumulate in the kidneys, where they cause continuous damage. For example, kidney-function loss is common among smokers, with tobacco toxins not only damaging the kidneys but also decreasing critical blood flow to the kidneys.

Another example is the heavy metal cadmium. Fortunately, the kidneys can quickly filter cadmium out of the blood. Unfortunately, the cadmium all too often gets stuck in the kidneys. Like many toxins, when concentrated, it damages these delicate tissues, causing oxidative stress. If you ever wonder what oxidation looks like in your body, all you need to do is look at a rusty car or at rubber that has cracked after being exposed to the sun for years. Rust is oxidized iron, and cracked rubber is oxidized carbon molecules. The same thing happens in your body, and it is especially significant when DNA or mitochondria are oxidized. These are the primary causes of aging.

The dramatic decline in our ability to get rid of toxins over time helps

Table 6.1. **Weeks 7 and 8 Foods and Supplements**

WEEKS 7 AND 8 FOODS
• No animal proteins (or dairy) during this week
• 3 ounces nuts and seeds like almonds, cashews, and pumpkin seeds (rich in magnesium) three times a day
• Two generous servings twice per day green leafy vegetables (rich in many nutrients) seasoned with dill and caraway
• One or two servings per day of a whole grain such as rice, millet, or quinoa
• Two citrus fruits (except grapefruit) twice a day
• Beet juice: 8 oz. twice a day
• Ginger juice, fresh: one inch a day, take with beet juice
• Blueberries: 1 cup a day
WEEKS 7 AND 8 SUPPLEMENTS
• Magnesium citrate: 500 mg twice a day
• Curcumin (either Theracurmin or Meriva): 300 mg twice a day
• Ginkgo biloba: 60 mg twice a day
• Gotu kola: 100 mg twice a day
• Fiber: 5 grams of a fiber supplement three times a day
• NAC: 500 mg three times a day
• A multivitamin
OTHER
• Decrease consumption of salt to less than ½ gram—approximately ⅛ tsp—per day (yes, you will find this surprisingly difficult).
• Decrease phosphates (for example, processed cheeses, canned fish, sunflower seeds) to less than 400 mg per day.
• Drink at least 4 quarts of clean, filtered water per day. (Carbon block filters work well!)
• Follow breathing instructions.

explain why almost everyone gets sicker with age. As you can see in figure 6.1, an eighty-five-year-old has only about half the kidney function of a twenty-year-old.

Protecting the Kidneys

The kidneys' principal task is filtering toxins from the blood. To do that job requires adequate blood flow through the kidneys, to ensure that the

Figure 6.1. **Deterioration in kidney function with aging**

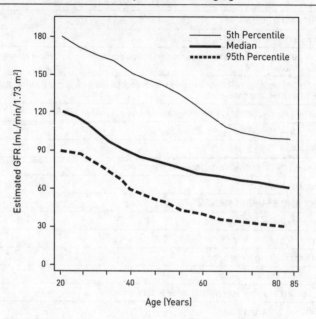

toxins can be cleared out. Only when there is sufficient microcirculation—the flow of blood through tiny blood vessels in the kidneys—can they perform effectively. Research now shows that impaired kidney blood flow may be the primary reason kidney function declines with aging.[2] Decreased blood flow also causes a buildup of scar tissue around the kidneys, which further decreases the amount of blood available for cleaning the kidneys.

Anything that lowers blood flow to the kidneys decreases the excretion of toxins. Smoking, elevated blood pressure, obesity, and even high-fat meals can damage microcirculation. While most people know that all of these aren't healthy, few are aware that certain widely used food additives seriously damage the kidneys' detoxification capacity by impairing microcirculation.

Figure 6.1 source: L. A. Frassetto, R. C. Morris Jr., and A. Sebastian, "Effect of age on blood acid-base composition in adult humans: Role of age-related renal functional decline," *American Journal of Physiology* 271, no. 6, pt. 2 (1996): F1114–22.

Three Ways the Kidneys Excrete Toxins

The kidneys get rid of toxins in the following three ways:

1. Filtration of most small and medium molecules from the blood. The glomerulus is like the strainer you use to drain pasta: it keeps the big molecules in the blood and allows the small molecules into the kidney for excretion in the urine, or, in the case of important molecules, for reabsorption back into the body.

2. Passive diffusion of fat-soluble molecules into the urine. Passive means that the toxins move by themselves from areas of high concentration, in the kidneys, to the urine, an area of lower concentration. Drinking sufficient water helps dilute the urine, making it easier for these toxins to leave the kidneys.

3. Active transport into the urine. This means the kidneys spend energy to create special enzymes and molecules to get particularly difficult toxins out of the blood and into the urine.

Figure 6.2. **Kidney filtration mechanism**

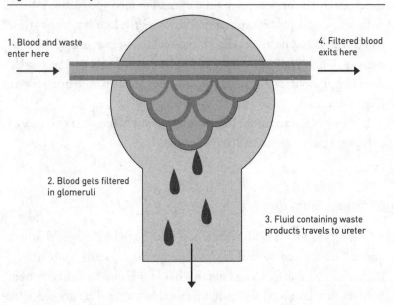

1. Blood and waste enter here

4. Filtered blood exits here

2. Blood gets filtered in glomeruli

3. Fluid containing waste products travels to ureter

Excessive Protein in the Diet

The average person should eat about 1 gram of protein per kilogram of body weight per day. So if you weigh 154 pounds (70 kilograms), you should eat 2⅓ ounces (70 grams) of protein a day. An egg is 6 grams of protein. Almost all natural foods have some protein, so you don't have to eat only high-protein foods. For example, 3 ounces of cabbage has 1 gram of protein. While high-protein diets can be effective for losing weight, following them for years at a time can be very hard on the kidneys.

Excessive Phosphates in the Diet

Phosphorus-containing additives, called phosphates, are used in myriad ways—for acid balancing, especially in carbonated beverages, leavening of bread, color and moisture retention, anticaking, and flavorings. Phosphorus is an essential mineral for cell structure and function, but when consumed in excess, it has many adverse effects.

When you consume foods, such as sodas, that contain high levels of phosphates, the phosphates eventually migrate into your bloodstream, where they can impair blood circulation to the kidneys, undermining the crucial filtration process so fundamental to successful detox.

Excessive phosphate consumption damages the kidneys, blocks their blood vessels, and decreases their filtration rate. In fact, one of the early signs of kidney failure is increasing phosphate levels in the blood.[3] Avoiding phosphates is difficult, because they are used in so many foods. (See table 6.2.)

In figure 6.3, you can see that excessive phosphorous intake is related to higher rates of mortality from all causes.

Charles's Story

As Charles aged, his health worsened. Although he thought that was normal, he noticed he had far less energy than friends his own age. Back when he was fifty years old, his blood pressure had already been quite elevated, indicating heart disease. He was also diagnosed with

Table 6.2. **Primary Sources of Phosphates**

PROCESSED FOOD TYPE	EXAMPLES OF PHOSPHATE ADDITIVES
Milk and dairy	Phosphoric acid, sodium phosphate, calcium phosphate, potassium tripolyphosphate
Mixed dishes, grain-based	Modified food starch, sodium acid pyrophosphate, disodium phosphate
Breads, rolls, and tortillas	Sodium aluminum phosphate, monocalcium phosphate, sodium acid pyrophosphate
Quick breads, bread products, sweet bakery products	Sodium acid pyrophosphate, sodium aluminum phosphate, monocalcium phosphate, dicalcium phosphate, calcium acid pyrophosphate
Poultry	Sodium tripolyphosphate, sodium tripoly / sodium hexa-metaphosphate blends, sodium acid pyrophosphate, tetrasodium pyrophosphate
Pizza	Disodium phosphate, tricalcium phosphate, tetrasodium pyrophosphate, sodium acid pyrophosphate
Vegetables	Monocalcium phosphate, sodium phosphate, disodium phosphate, sodium acid pyrophosphate, disodium hydrogen pyrophosphate
Mixed dishes: meat, poultry, seafood	Sodium tripolyphosphate, sodium acid pyrophosphate, tricalcium phosphate, trisodium phosphate
Meats	Potassium tripolyphosphate, tetrapotassium pyrophosphate, sodium hexametaphosphate
Plant-based protein foods	Sodium hexametaphosphate, sodium tripolyphosphate
Cereals	Disodium phosphate, tricalcium phosphate, trisodium phosphate
Eggs	Sodium hexametaphosphate, potassium tripolyphosphate, monosodium phosphate
Seafood	Sodium acid pyrophosphate, potassium tripolyphosphate, tetrapotassium pyrophosphate, sodium tripolyphosphate
Savory snacks, crackers, snack /meal bars	Calcium phosphate, sodium hexametaphosphate, tricalcium phosphate
Other desserts	Calcium phosphate, modified corn starch, disodium phosphate, tetrasodium pyrophosphate
Sugar sweetened / diet beverages /alcoholic beverages	Phosphoric acid
100% juice	Calcium phosphate
Fruits	Monopotassium phosphate
Soups	Disodium phosphate, tricalcium phosphate
Condiments, sauces	Phosphoric acid, disodium phosphate, modified food starch, sodium hexamonophosphate

Table 6.2 source: Adapted from M. S. Calvo, A. J. Moshfegh, and K. L. Tucker, "Assessing the health impact of phosphorus in the food supply: Issues and considerations," *Advances in Nutrition* 5, no. 1 (2014): 104–13.

Figure 6.3. **Excessive phosphorus intake and its contribution to all-cause mortality**

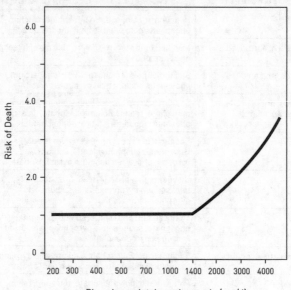

Phosphorus Intake on log-scale (mg/d)

type 2 diabetes. Now that he was sixty-one, he felt so chronically ill that his doctor ran more extensive laboratory tests and determined that Charles had declining kidney function. Further testing showed damage and blockage of the arteries leading to his kidneys. His filtration rate was very poor, like that of a ninety-year-old man. His plasma creatinine (a waste product of muscle metabolism) was elevated as well, since the kidneys are responsible for its excretion. His kidney specialist predicted he would need to go on dialysis within eighteen to twenty-four months.

My colleague Kerry Bone, an expert herbalist from Australia, recommended that Charles go on a three-part program—one nearly identical

Figure 6.3 source: A. R. Chang, M. Lazo, L. J. Appel, O. M. Gutiérrez, and M. E. Grams, "High dietary phosphorus intake is associated with all-cause mortality: Results from NHANES III," *American Journal of Clinical Nutrition* 99, no. 2 (2014): 320–27.

to what you will follow during the second week of this phase of the Toxin Solution. On the program, Charles ate more nitrate-rich foods (green leafy vegetables and beet juice) and decreased inflammation by eating chocolate, blueberries, raspberries, strawberries, blackberries, and garlic. The primary supplements he took—fish oil, turmeric, and anthocyanins—also worked to decrease inflammation. The main herbal medicines on the program were ginger, gotu kola, and ginkgo biloba to improve microcirculation. Five months later, Charles returned for a reevaluation. Many kidney measures, including filtration, had improved dramatically.

Results like his are simply unheard of in conventional medicine, where kidney failure is always considered progressive. Months later, Charles was *not* on dialysis, and his filtration rate was like that of a fifty-year-old man.

The bottom line is that when the kidneys don't function well, people can't successfully detoxify. But that trend can be reversed. Relentless progressive loss of kidney function may be the norm, but it is certainly not inevitable. Thanks to following the protocol, the toxin filtration rate of Charles's kidneys doubled, from 35 to 74—an improvement unheard of in conventional medicine. He experienced a steady improvement in health and well-being. Giving your body a chance to heal means stopping the damage and facilitating regeneration.

So how about you? Do you want the kidneys of someone many years older or of someone many years younger?

Improving Microcirculation

What can you do to improve your kidneys' detoxification capacity? Since sufficient blood flow through the kidneys is so critical to detoxification, on this plan you will consume foods, herbs, and spices known to benefit kidney microcirculation. As you will notice, most of the items I recommend are widely available. Many of them are delicious. Undertaking this program is no hardship and conveys so many benefits. Over the next two weeks, please include in your daily nutrition as many of the following as possible:

- Beetroot juice
- Blueberries
- Chocolate
- Curcumin (turmeric)

- Ginkgo biloba
- Ginger
- Gotu kola
- A multivitamin

Beetroot Juice

On this plan, you will drink eight ounces of freshly juiced beets, twice a day. Beetroot juice is brimming with naturally occurring nitrates, which convert to nitric oxide when you eat or drink them. Nitric oxide dilates the blood vessels, leading to significantly increased blood flow. One study found that beetroot juice greatly improves the distance people with peripheral vascular disease can walk before they experience severe pain—evidence of its ability to improve circulation by dilating blood vessels. (See figure 6.4.)

Figure 6.4. **Walking time in minutes until pain is experienced**

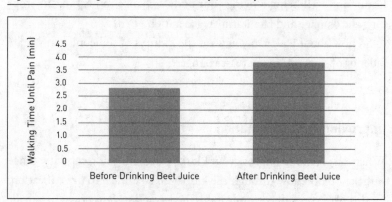

Figure 6.4 source: Adapted from A. A. Kenjale, K. L. Ham, T. Stabler, et al., "Dietary nitrate sup-plementation enhances exercise performance in peripheral arterial disease," *Journal of Applied Physiology* 110, no. 6 (2011): 1582–91.

Since one of the goals in reviving the kidneys is increasing microcirculation, you can see the extraordinary benefit of drinking beet juice for the kidneys.

Chocolate

Dark chocolate (choose the low- or no-sugar version with at least 65 percent cacao) also supports the kidneys by improving oxygenation and increasing blood flow to the kidneys.[4] Other substances in chocolate, such as catechins, protect the kidneys from oxidative stress and from certain toxic drugs.[5]

Blueberries

Blueberries are close to a miracle drug. In chapter 4, I discussed how gut toxins damage the kidneys. Blueberries slightly increase the filtration rate in normal kidneys, while also protecting them from the dramatic lowering of the filtration rate caused by gut toxins.

Curcumin (Turmeric)

If you're looking for even more reasons to eat curries, drink turmeric tea, and supplement with the Indian spice turmeric, curcumin (the active ingredient in turmeric) protects the kidneys from toxins, maintains filtration rates, and protects against cadmium.

Ginkgo Biloba

Ask any Western natural medicine practitioner what herb best improves circulation, and most will recommend *ginkgo biloba*—shown to improve blood supply in the brain and in other critical tissues. One study found that ginkgo improves kidney blood flow and function.[6]

An important study showed that ginkgo also effectively protects the kidneys from glyphosate, a common herbicide used in GMO agriculture that is especially toxic to the kidneys.[7] Other animal studies have shown that ginkgo protects kidneys from mercury, uranium, naphthalene, and many other toxins.[8] You will take ginkgo daily during the Two-Week Kidney Detox Protocol.

Ginger

During these two weeks, you will benefit from drinking ginger tea, using ginger to spice foods, and taking ginger supplements (if you wish). Although human studies have yet to catch up to animal studies, there's plenty of research indicating that ginger both improves kidney function and protects the kidneys from cadmium. One study found that the anti-inflammatory effects of ginger were so strong, it was able to prevent most of the cadmium damage to the kidneys.[9] Ginger's anti-inflammatory benefits derive from its antioxidant properties, along with its ability to tune down pro-inflammatory genes.[10] Another study found that ginger specifically increases the activity of the kidneys' own antioxidant enzymes.

One animal study showed that ginger strongly protects from alcohol toxicity, while another showed that it protects from a pesticide.[11] Many studies show that ginger protects the kidneys from carbon tetrachloride, chromates, fructose, gentamicin, ischemia, lead, cancer drugs, and other toxins.

Gotu Kola

Gotu kola has been used in Chinese traditional medicine to treat kidney diseases for a very long time. It improves microcirculation and reverses fibrosis (the thickening and scarring of connective tissue). Research suggests that gotu kola also offers protection from toxic drugs.[12] Another study combined gotu kola with naringenin (from grapefruit) and showed that together they blocked the scar-tissue formation that decreases blood flow and causes so much damage in kidneys.[13]

Multivitamin

Finally, be sure to take a good-quality multivitamin and mineral supplement. I am not looking here for high dosages, but rather as many nutrients as possible, at around two times the recommended daily allowance (RDA).

Water

While detoxing, it's vital to decrease the stress on your kidneys by drinking three to four quarts of clean water per day. *Clean water* means either distilled water, water that is bottled in glass, or water that is filtered through a carbon block filter or reverse osmosis. This helps keep the toxins diluted as they move through your system, especially your kidneys. This is not about drinking as much as you can. You can overload your kidneys with too much water.

Alkalinizing Your Tissues

The program outlined at the beginning of this chapter (page 177) will both decrease the toxic load on your kidneys and stimulate circulation and filtration. Key to this program is that some toxins are best excreted when the urine is more alkaline and others are best eliminated when the urine is more acid. Fortunately, you can control the acid–alkaline balance. Although there are many subtleties to this, eating a protein-rich diet will tend to acidify your urine, while consuming a diet with plentiful fruits and vegetables will tend to alkalinize your urine. Since virtually everyone is way too acidic, during weeks 7 and 8, on this plan, you will emphasize alkalinizing your urine by eating the foods and taking the supplements I recommend.

In order to further facilitate your body's alkalinity, you can continue to take mineral citrates. At least a gram a day of magnesium plus potassium citrates is the recommended dose. This will give you two solid weeks of alkalinizing.

To accomplish that, as much as possible eat organically grown food (see the Dirty Dozen [page 74] and Clean 15 [page 99]), with your meals prepared low in salt and phosphates and high in fiber.

Another method for alkalinizing the system is to use a specific breathing exercise. This breathing pattern will result in your exhaling more carbon dioxide than usual—another way of getting acid out of the body.

When you breathe, you exhale carbon dioxide. This results in slight alkalinization of the blood. When deeper breathing is continued for several minutes at a time, the cells, pericellular spaces (the spaces surrounding a cell), and kidneys become more alkaline, resulting in an increased excretion of toxins. Breathing calmly and slowly does not mean hyperventilating. Too much breathing can be as much of a problem as too little. During this week, you need to consciously breathe more deeply more often. Rather than recommend a specific breathing protocol, I suggest you go to one of the many yoga websites that provide recommendations on safe deep breathing. Some may wonder if "alkaline water" would help here. Unfortunately I could not find any solid research that addressed this important question.

Review of Kidney Cleanse

In sum, during these two weeks, decrease salt and phosphates; drink plenty of clean water; eat leafy green vegetables, blueberries, raspberries, citrus fruits, beet juice, gotu kola, ginkgo biloba, ginger, and curcumin; and engage daily in the breathing exercises.

Remember, if toxins are being released too quickly, you will feel sicker and your vitality will be lower. If you have especially high levels of some specific toxins, it can even be dangerous. This is very unlikely, but the risk is not zero. An extreme example is what happened in Japan to people living in the city of Minamata. Due to high levels of highly toxic industrial methyl mercury released into a river where people fished, the population had a lot of neurological disease. When they lost weight—for whatever reason—their neurological symptoms got much worse because the body could not get rid of the mercury fast enough.

Your health is in your hands, and by protecting your kidneys with foods, herbs, and spices that support microcirculation and other kidney functions, you can markedly improve your kidneys' capacity to detox your blood.

7

Intense Full-Body Detox

Now that you have cleansed and activated the body's three major detox organs, you are ready for a final week's full detoxification. This is pretty intense and entirely optional, but if you feel like you really want to go for it, here's what you can do. I recommend that you do this if at all possible, because now that your detoxification system is functioning optimally, you have a unique opportunity to rid your body of even more deeply buried toxins, ones that you could never before access and release.

Although some readers may be tempted, I counsel you *not* to jump in and undertake this program without first following the protocols in the prior eight weeks. The reason? Again, you must prepare your organs—and do it in the right sequence—in order to detox safely.

Sending Your Body the Right Signals

For a more active detox, there are certain ways to "tell your body" that it's time to intensify your detox. Since your liver, kidneys, hair, and skin are always getting rid of the toxins in your blood, you need to amp up the

messages to the cells and the fluids between your cells to start releasing.
During this week you will send those messages by:

- Decreasing the number of calories you are consuming

- Continuing an alkaline diet—by limiting animal protein and
  consuming lots of fruits and vegetables

- Sweating out toxins through taking saunas

- Drinking green drinks

- Releasing toxins from the lymph system through massage

The diet that you started following in chapter 6 is alkaline. Now I'll
show you how to up the ante, should you choose to.

Caloric Restriction

In this, the final week of the Nine-Week Toxin Solution, you may slightly
reduce your caloric intake by eating nutrient-dense, low-calorie foods.
Although the mild calorie restriction you will undergo during this final
week is highly beneficial, many people avoid undertaking a detox (or
fast) because they fear being hungry. Yes, assuring adequate nourishment
is fundamental to survival. Yet with the current barrage of bad food, an
active hunger trigger isn't the survival advantage it once was.

Processed foods, designed to seduce our taste buds, easily trigger hunger, leading people to eat bad food. Nearly one-third of our population
is obese, suffering from a host of ensuing health problems. Getting used
to feeling slightly hungry during week 9 is not life endangering, it's life
prolonging.

Over the millennia that we evolved as a species, food was not always
available. People who could not endure temporary food unavailability
died out. But the rest of humankind evolved. When people burn fat
for calories, the body releases ketones into the blood. Ketones cause
mood elevation when they reach the brain, ensuring that you don't
mope around, fail to take appropriate action, and die from starvation

when you're hungry. Instead, you are genetically designed to function even with reduced calorie intake. The benefits to calorie restriction are increased longevity and decreased chronic disease burden. The animal research may apply to humans as well. The life-span-increasing effects of caloric restriction were first shown in fruit flies. (Fruit flies are easy to study because they have a short life span.) This research has now been reproduced in one of our close relatives, the rhesus monkey. Restricting the monkeys' calories increased average longevity from twenty-six to thirty years—a remarkable 15 percent increase in life span![1]

How to Restrict Your Calories

Begin by keeping a food diary for three days prior to launching week 9 of the plan. Please note exactly what you eat, and consult any of the many available apps to easily determine your current calorie baseline. Whatever your baseline, dial it down until you are consuming five hundred to one thousand fewer calories a day than previously. (This assumes your weight was stable. If you were gaining weight, you'll need to restrict calories more.) This means about one thousand calories for an average woman and fifteen hundred for an average man. Remember, your goal is not losing weight—although you will—but rather balancing your release rate with your elimination capability.

Caloric restriction, along with the other features of this plan, sends your body the message that it's "time to detox." The lower your calorie count, the quicker the detox process. I have supervised many water fasts and am a great believer in fasting's benefits. Nevertheless, accelerating detox (through caloric restriction or fasting) is safest to do only after all the detox organs have been prepared. For those who fear or dislike fasting, simply reducing calorie intake is a safe and practicable way to experience many of its benefits.

By adjusting your calorie consumption, you adjust the rate of detox. If possible, do this for the final week to harvest the full benefits of the Toxin Solution.

Saunas

Many cultures recognize the value of saunas, but one of their prime benefits is detoxification. Without necessarily knowing that, in cultures as diverse as the Native American, Finnish, and Japanese, people have experienced the same feeling of vitality that most people feel today after a good, long sauna. The research has now clarified the reasons: sweating is excellent at getting toxins of all classes out of our body.

Roger's Story

A normally gentle and friendly giant, Roger had become increasingly irritable recently. I learned this when his wife, Sheila, brought him to me. The day before, Roger had become furious over some trifle and had thrust his fist through a wall in their home. Sheila felt frightened that he might hurt her and their children. Had the family been unknown to me, I might have called social services. However, in this case I knew Roger, and was myself surprised to hear of this change in him. I began to investigate further.

Roger owned a small home-construction company. The firm was growing, but Roger did a lot of the work himself rather than subcontracting to others. While his primary skill was carpentry, he was now also doing fine cabinetry, plumbing, electrical work, and painting. At this point in my practice, I was now suspecting that anyone with disease might be suffering from toxicity. Roger's exposure to solvents from the cabinetry varnish and metals released from the copper pipes he installed, along with chemicals from the drying paints, all resulted in a substantial toxic load. Solvents are highly toxic chemicals that can cause damage to the liver, kidneys, and nervous system. The good news is that we are pretty good at detoxifying solvents. The bad news is that we can be constantly exposed to them.

But Roger was unwilling to follow my suggestions. Stop exposure to toxins? Nope. Hire someone else to do it? Nope. Well, you get the idea.

He would not take herbs or vitamins, and he thought hydrotherapy was a joke. I don't know why I thought of it, but in desperation I asked if he liked saunas.

He smiled. It turned out that his wife had asked him to build one for their home, but he had been too busy with the paying customers. He then sheepishly apologized for being so rude and admitted that even he feared for his family when he got so angry. He decided to get together with his team and quickly built a nice sauna for their home. He then faithfully used the sauna for one hour every day, sweating profusely. As he began to release his toxic burden, he also relented and agreed to make his workplace safer so that he could avoid taking in additional toxins. Within a week, he felt noticeably better, and within a month he was back to his normal self.

The scientific literature shows the range of toxins excreted by saunas. In general, the concentration of most toxins is two to ten times higher in sweat than in blood, clearly indicating that the body is effectively utilizing sweating as a significant detoxification process.[2]

Table 7.1. **Detoxification Through Saunas**

CATEGORY	EXAMPLES
Toxic metals	Arsenic, cadmium, lead, mercury
Persistent organic pollutants	Polybrominated biphenyls (PBBs), polychlorinated biphenyls (PCBs), phthalates and phthalate metabolites (DMP, DEP, DBP, BBP, DCHP, DEHP, and DINP), perfluorinated compounds (PFHxS, PFOS, PFOA, and PFNA)
Solvents and small molecules	Methamphetamine, solvents
Other benefits	Increases lipolysis; increases production of growth hormone

It may interest you to know that even police and firefighters are using saunas for health reasons. A big health hazard for law-enforcement personnel comes from repeated exposure to methamphetamine and related production chemical compounds when they raid meth labs. With frequent exposure, the police officers, firefighters, and social workers develop chronic symptoms, some so severe that they become disabled. Research suggests that half of law-enforcement personnel involved in this type of enforcement work develop varying degrees of chronic illness, symptoms, and disability. If you have ever had to deal with a meth addict, you can readily understand how bad this drug is for health.

For this severely exposed group, saunas every day for a month dramatically lowered their toxic load and decreased their symptoms 70 to 90 percent, allowing almost all to return to work.[3] If you have no access to a sauna, use a stationary bicycle, and exercise hard enough to sweat. Again, it does not matter *how* you sweat, just as long as you sweat a lot and get rid of the toxins leaving your body as quickly as possible. In the instructions that follow, I'll help you detox using a sauna safely and effectively.

The Best Way to Take Saunas

How often should you do a sauna? It depends upon how heavy a toxic load you have built up. I am not suggesting you take one every day, but every other day would be good.

Obviously, the best place for a sauna is at home, where you can do it by yourself, without exposure to other people's toxins. If possible, open the window a crack so you can allow in fresh air while the contaminants evaporate from your skin and lungs and circulate out the window. Sit on towels and wash them thoroughly. The type of sauna does not matter; all that counts is that you sweat profusely. If, unlike Roger, you don't have a home sauna, use one at a gym, but try to do so at times when no one else is in the sauna. I don't recommend steam baths, since the steam will recirculate the toxins.

If you aren't used to saunas, start at a lower temperature and work your way up slowly. Your goal is to sweat profusely for at least thirty minutes.

The key to optimizing your benefit from saunas is to get the temperature, duration, and hydration balanced properly. Ultimately, you should be perspiring in a way that releases an oily sweat. Here's how you can achieve that.

The first day, start at 110 degrees Fahrenheit for fifteen minutes. If you start sweating within five minutes and are sweating heavily by ten minutes, this is the right temperature for you. If not, increase the temperature to 120 degrees the next time you take a sauna. If you aren't heavily sweating within ten minutes, increase the temperature to 130 degrees. You should sweat profusely. Once you determine the right temperature—the one that prompts you to sweat heavily within ten minutes—stay in the sauna for at least thirty minutes after you started.

Don't overdo it. If you are really toxic, or if your physiological system is not yet strong enough, you can't use as high a temperature or stay in as long.

When you use saunas to get rid of toxins, always replenish the trace minerals lost in your sweat.[4] While many people think of replenishing only salt, the reality is that *all* trace minerals are lost. There are several ways to do this: through the green drinks I recommend in the next section, or by taking a good-quality trace-mineral supplement every day.

Weigh yourself before and after to assure that you are consuming enough fluids. If you lose weight, add an additional volume of fluids to match the weight you lost. For example, if you lost one pound, you need to consume an extra two cups of water. With every two cups of water, take a trace-mineral supplement.

Finally, if you have any serious disease, such as heart failure, cardiac arrhythmia, chronic obstructive pulmonary disease (COPD), uncontrolled high blood pressure, or poorly controlled diabetes, you *must* first check with your doctor before using a sauna. Saunas during pregnancy are definitely not advised until after at least the first trimester. Also, no alcohol! This ought to be obvious, since you are trying to detoxify. Although sauna deaths are extremely rare, when they do occur, 44 percent are due to alcohol consumption.[5]

Green Drinks

Vegetable juices are rich in trace minerals, helping to replenish those you lose in the saunas. Green drinks made from green tea and vegetables, especially vegetables from the cabbage family, are also very effective in upregulating Phase I and Phase II liver-detoxification enzymes.[6] In addition, their high level of antioxidants protect cells from the toxins being released. I recommend a pint a day, but be careful to avoid too much green tea, since the caffeine it contains can make you jittery, which you don't want.

You can either make a green drink yourself or buy a premade product. Green drinks are easy to make if you have a juicer or blender. I prefer machines that keep the pulp with the juice, since the fiber is an important part of the detoxification process. Be sure you buy plenty of organically grown greens; you may be quite surprised by how much is needed for a full glass.

While fresh is best, it does take some work, and cleaning up can be a hassle. If you prefer a more convenient solution, premade green drinks are very convenient. But please be sure you buy from a reputable, high-quality company. There are a number of good products available. Two that I like are Enriching Blueberry Greens, by Natural Factors (full disclosure: I consult for their health-care professional product line) and Pure Synergy Superfood, by the Synergy Company. I have carefully inspected the manufacturing facilities of both companies and use their products myself.

Massage

Since our interstitial spaces and lymphatics contain a lot of toxins, a good-quality massage will help drain these out more quickly. I could not find any direct research, but I did find some that certainly supports the importance of massage. Several studies have shown that when infants with jaundice are massaged, the bilirubin that turns them yellow is eliminated 20 percent more quickly after just four days of twice-daily twenty-minute massage.[7] Clearly the massage is getting the bilirubin in the tissues back into circulation so it can be better eliminated. Despite the paucity of research, I've found that massage is very helpful with my own patients in decreasing their discomfort while detoxifying. That is why during this final week, I recommend that you get a massage one to three times.

Conclusion

You have now completed the Nine-Week Toxin Solution. You have accomplished a lot: avoided toxins where you can, altered your diet, and cleansed and strengthened your body's three main organs of detox-ification. Finally, you capped that off with a week of intensified toxin release through caloric restriction and sweating out toxins, supported by the added nutritional boost of green drinks, along with massage to release any toxins stored in your lymphatic system and interstitial spaces. Although you may have felt a little rocky at times during the detox, by now you should be feeling a lot better than you have been in a long time.

Congratulations on completing the program. The improved energy, better sleep, and greater stamina and resilience that you now experience are a testament to your body's rejuvenative capacity. This is a program that you can also repeat periodically. I recommend undertaking it three to four times per year. While most of the program can safely be followed during your regular life, week 9 is a great one to do if you have a break or vacation. Because the caloric restriction makes this week resemble a mini-fast, it's a wonderful opportunity to rest and complete your recovery.

Remember: although you have taken a break from toxins, the toxins themselves are still out there in our world. How can you maintain and build on what you have accomplished?

The next chapter answers this question.

8

Stay Healthy and Detoxed

Because this is an age when chemical and industrial toxins are so pervasive, the threats to health are also unprecedented. Earlier eras had to deal with sudden death from infections and accidents that people now recover from easily with the help of surgery or antibiotics. But advances in modern technology and science have left us with another problem—the accumulating effects of toxicity. The slow accrual of harmful chemicals in your body can gradually erode your organs and systems and lead to chronic disease.

I believe you have followed the Toxin Solution because you want to protect yourself from this outcome. And the good news, as you found out from reading this book so far, is that it is possible. Even in our toxic world. Now the challenge is to maintain and consolidate those gains. In this chapter, I show you how to maintain your progress going forward, following the new baseline for health you've established. While continuing to limit your exposure to toxins, you will learn how to maintain a healthy diet and lifestyle. You will learn how to ensure that your body deals efficiently with the toxins you cannot avoid. At the end of the chapter, I will describe how to use the information in the book's appendices to test your own toxic load and to access longer-term treatments, if needed.

The Toxin Solution Maintenance Plan

There are three goals to my Toxin Solution Maintenance Plan:

1. Keep new toxins from entering your body.

2. Keep decreasing your toxic load.

3. Improve key functions of your physiology so you can live a long and healthy life.

Here I will focus on the first two of these three keys to maintenance—keeping toxins out and decreasing your toxic load. The third is a topic for another book. (My 1996 book *Total Wellness* is now a bit out-of-date but fully addresses how to optimize all aspects of your physiology.)

Keep Out New Toxins

The Toxin Solution began by examining the causes of toxic overload, and what you can do about it. I want to reemphasize an important point I made in those earlier chapters: Although many toxins cannot be readily avoided, it is *much* easier to avoid the avoidable toxins than it is to get them out of your body. It takes months to years, in many cases, to get just half the amount of many of these poisons out of your body. Obviously, you can't hold your breath to avoid inhaling polluted air, nor can you easily avoid medications that people flushed away and therefore have found their way into many regional and municipal water supplies. But as I showed you in chapters 2 and 3, you can avoid many kinds of avoidable toxins—so please make sure you do.

Some of the recommendations I make in this chapter may be expensive. Rather than advising you repeatedly to undertake these steps "if you can afford them," I simply make the suggestion, and you can determine which approaches you can afford. Occasionally, I will also suggest less expensive alternatives.

After reading the Detox Maintenance Protocol and the explanations that follow it, you may wonder if the maintenance program is excessive. I don't think it is. My own family has decided that ongoing detox is so important to our health that we do virtually everything I recommend here. Yes, the list is long—but the truth is, it could be even longer.

Sadly, as I discussed in chapter 2, the major source of toxins is the food we eat every day. I recommend the following practices when either growing, purchasing, cooking, or storing your food.

Eat Organically Grown Food

Many foods are contaminated during their growing or processing or from the containers in which they are stored. That is why I recommend that you eat only organically grown foods—and store your food properly (in glass). I realize the sticker shock people experience due to the prices of organic food. That is why many people I know have joined a food cooperative or subscribed to a CSA (community-supported agriculture) in order to keep their organic food costs down. There are an increasing number of food co-ops and CSAs across the country. Food co-ops, particularly worker-operated food co-ops, offer the added benefit of opening the door to a community of health-minded people like yourself. If you can't afford to eat everything organically grown or you must eat in restaurants frequently, be sure to at least avoid eating the foods on the Dirty Dozen Plus Two list (see page 74)—fourteen foods that should be eaten only if they are organically grown.

Avoid Additives and Preservatives

As I have been cautioning throughout *The Toxin Solution*, read food labels and avoid foods that, despite the "natural" label claims, are filled with

204   THE TOXIN SOLUTION

Table 8.1. **Detox Maintenance Protocol**

Food	• Eat organically grown, unprocessed food. • Avoid foods with additives and synthetic preservatives. • Grow some of your own food. • Do not buy food packaged in plastic or use plastic for storing food. • Avoid aluminum and Teflon cookware. • Limit barbecued, grilled, and charbroiled foods. • Limit alcohol consumption. If you do drink, wine and beer are "best" and aged liquors are worst. • Use the least toxic forms of marijuana if this is a drug of your choice.
Air	• Install HEPA air filters in your home. • Avoid ozone machines and wood fireplaces, since they release unhealthy oxidizing compounds. • Change the filters on your heating and cooling systems regularly.
Water	• Filter the water you use for cooking and bathing.
Household and yard	• Use carbon monoxide alarms and nonradioactive smoke alarms. • Use fragrance-free natural household cleansers low in solvents, or make your own. • Clean, dust, and vacuum regularly. • Avoid "Scotchgard"-ing your furniture. • Check for black mold in any potentially wet area of your home periodically. • Wear natural fibers. • Use nontoxic paints. • Use bedding materials made from natural products with no or low release of VOCs (volatile organic compounds).
Health and beauty aids	• Use natural products without fragrance that are low in chemicals and free of phthalates.
Additional detoxing	• Continue eating cabbage-family foods. • Continue taking fiber supplements. • Use a sauna periodically, or exercise, to generate sweating.

added chemicals. The longer the list of ingredients, the more likely it is that there is something in the food that's bad for your health. The list of top preservatives and additives to be on the lookout for is long.

Note that this list includes salt and phosphates, as well as the many synthetic preservatives and flavor enhancers. And don't be fooled by such claims as "Nothing artificial added." This can be very misleading, because the food product manufacturers have their raw-material suppliers add the noxious chemicals beforehand, so they can say they themselves didn't. Look for the "USDA Certified Organic" label instead.

Table 8.2. **Preservatives and Additives**

CHEMICAL	WHAT IT DOES	WHERE IT'S FOUND
Acacia gum	Stabilizer	Soft drink syrups, gummy candies, marshmallows, M&M's, chocolate candies, edible glitter
Ammonium sulfate	To activate baking yeast	Baked goods
Artificial colors, anything beginning with FD&C	Adds color to make poor-quality foods look better	Most colorful processed foods
Aspartame, acesulfame-K, saccharin	Artificial sweeteners	Artificially sweetened foods, especially soft drinks, and in packets at restaurants
Benzoyl peroxide	Bleaching agent	White flour
Butylated hydroxyanisole (BHA)	Synthetic antioxidant	Packaged foods, baked goods
Butylated hydroxytoluene (BHT) or butylhydroxytoluene	Synthetic antioxidants	Packaged foods, baked goods
Calcium, potassium, or sodium propionates	Mold inhibitors	Processed foods
Carnauba wax (palm or Brazil wax)	Coating and glazing	Hard candies
Carrageenan	Thickening agent	Creamy foods and desserts
Castoreum	"Natural" flavoring	As a substitute for vanilla
Corn syrup; high-fructose corn syrup	Sweetener	Almost all sweetened processed foods
Cyclamate and cyclamic acid	Artificial sweeteners	Artificially sweetened foods
Dextrose	Sweetener	Desserts, sweets, cookies, candy
Diphenyl, biphenyl	Preservatives	Citrus fruits
Disodium ribonucleotides, inosinate, and guanylate	Flavor enhancers	Any foods with MSG
Dodecyl gallate	Synthetic antioxidant	Packaged foods
Heptylparaben	Preservative	Cosmetics
Hexamine, hexamethylene, tetramine	Preservatives	Caviar, cheese, herring, and preserved fish
Hydrogenated vegetable oil and partially hydrogenated vegetable oil	Preservatives	"Chewy" foods
Insoluble polyvinylpyrrolidone	Stabilizer and clarifying agent added to wine, beer, medications, pharmaceuticals	Shampoo, toothpaste, white wine, beer
Mannitol	Artificial sweetener	Sugar-free mint candies and gums
Monosodium glutamate (MSG) and all glutamates	Flavor enhancers	Many processed foods
Octyl gallate	Synthetic antioxidant	Cosmetics, perfume, soap, shampoo

CHEMICAL	WHAT IT DOES	WHERE IT'S FOUND
Olestra	Fat substitute	Pringles Light
Orthophenyl	Preservative	Citrus fruits
Paraffin, Vaseline, white mineral oil	Solvents, coating and glazing, antifoaming agents, lubricants	Shiny foods
Phosphates	Balance food acidity	Many processed foods
Polyoxyethylene sorbitan monostearate	Emulsifiers, stabilizers, gelling, thickening agents	See Polysorbate
Polysorbate	Emulsifier	Any food with water and oil kept in suspension
Potassium acesulfame	Sweetener	Sugar-free baked goods
Potassium and sodium nitrate	Preservatives	Cured meats
Potassium bromate	Flour bleaching	Baked goods (this is really important as competes with iodine and causes low thyroid)
Potassium ferrocyanide	Anticaking agent	Table salt (some sea salt as well)
Potassium nitrate	Preservative	Preserved meat
Propyl gallate	Synthetic antioxidant	Cosmetics with oils
Quinoline yellow	Food dye	Yellow processed foods
Saccharin	Sweetener	Sugar-free foods, packets at restaurants
Salt	Taste enhancer	Virtually all processed foods
Sodium and potassium bisulfite	Preservatives, bleaching agents	Prepared salads, dried fruits, wine
Sodium carboxymethyl cellulose	Viscosity modifier, thickener	Toothpaste, laxatives, diet pills, water-based paints, detergents, textile sizing, paper products
Sodium, potassium, and calcium sulfite	Preservatives	See Bisulfites above
Sulfur dioxide	Preservative	Dried fruits
Tartrazine	Food coloring	Yellow processed foods
Tert butylhydroquinone (TBHQ)	Synthetic antioxidant	Vegetable and animal fats
Titanium dioxide	Pigment, opacifier, sunscreen	Foods with artificial white pigments

Table 8.2 sources: Modified from www.traditionaloven.com/articles/122/dangerous-food-additives-to-avoid; www.sheknows.com/food-and-recipes/articles/960469/top-10-preservatives-and-additives-to-avoid.

Grow Some of Your Own Food

While writing this book, I happened to have dinner at a conference with one of my top graduates, Dr. Gaetano Morello, who practices in Vancouver, British Columbia. He made a comment that really resonated with me: "I have noticed that every one of my patients who is aging well has their own food garden. I think this helps them not only due to freshness and lack of pesticides, but the natural bacteria in the soil appears to promote a healthier gut."

If you are able to do so, grow at least some of your own food. If you do start a garden, use only natural fertilizers and sprays when needed. And avoid pesticides on your lawn as well: you don't want to breathe these chemicals or track them into your house. Do not include supposedly organic recycled city grass clippings in your compost or food garden. Urban grass is often grown with high-phosphate fertilizers that are contaminated with cadmium. As already discussed, this extremely toxic bluish-white metal has made its way into the food supply. Also, don't spray weed killers like Roundup anywhere on your property, since it can also get into your food.

Do Not Buy Food Packaged in Plastic

Pay attention to how your food is packaged, cooked, and stored. Do not buy food in packages with plastic or waxed liners. The chemicals used to make plastic nonsticky, malleable, and soft can contain phthalates and BPA. These known endocrine disruptors can negatively affect cardiovascular health by raising your blood pressure and can affect your energy by decreasing thyroid hormone production. While you're at it, get rid of all the plastic containers you use to store food at home—in the refrigerator, freezer, and pantry.

When you buy condiments like mustard and ketchup, or peanut and other nut butters, choose the ones in the glass jars instead of the plastic. That not only is healthier for you but will also provide you with good storage jars once you have consumed the product. Wash and save the jars and their lids for storing food. If you find that the lids are plastic, make sure not to overfill these jars so as to keep the food out of contact with the lid.

Plastic in lids often contains BPA (bisphenol A). No, I am not being OCD here—every source of exposure adds up. Anytime you can avoid a toxin, you should do so, because there are so many toxins we can't avoid.

When purchasing containers, look for ones made of borosilicate glass or soda-lime glass, which behave like Pyrex and can withstand heat and cold. If you absolutely must use canned goods or plastic, make sure they are BPA-free.

Avoid Teflon and Aluminum Cookware

For some time, there have been concerns about the use of aluminum cookware. Because aluminum is extremely soft, it leaches into the food that is cooked in it. High amounts of this metal have been found in the brain tissues of those with Alzheimer's disease. My best assessment of the research suggests that aluminum is not a significant cause of dementia—but it causes other problems. This is why it is now banned in many countries, including Germany, France, Great Britain, Switzerland, Argentina, and Brazil. Use stainless steel, cast iron, or ceramic.

And get rid of your Teflon pots and pans once and for all. If you can't or don't want to lose your favorite Teflon fry pan, then learn how to use it correctly: never let it get hotter than 350 degrees. The problem is that you are not only cooking with Teflon, but *eating* Teflon (polyfluorotetraethylene) as well! This coating breaks apart at high heat, and can cause flu-like symptoms known as *Teflon flu*. Polyfluorotetraethylene has been linked in some studies with low birth weight, elevated cholesterol, abnormal thyroid hormone levels, liver inflammation, and weakened immune defense.

Recommended Cooking Techniques

It's healthier to steam, stir-fry, bake, or stew your food. Avoid cooking food at high temperatures without first protecting the food from air. When proteins, fats, or carbohydrates are cooked at high temperatures in the presence of oxygen, they form toxic and carcinogenic substances.

There are a number of ways to do this. I strongly recommend you look at the "healthy stir-fry" described on the World's Healthiest Foods website (www.WHFoods.org). My team of nutritionists and I worked with George Mateljan to determine the best ways to cook foods so the nutrients would be most available and the least damage would be done to the food. Basically, the trick is to use a small amount of water rather than oil in your cooking pan. For desired taste, oil can be added after cooking. This keeps the food from getting too hot and the oil from being damaged.

Limit Alcohol Consumption

If you are going to drink alcohol, consume the least toxic types. For example, wine made from "old vine" grapes has a lot more arsenic, which is used to keep down mold. Organic wine is better, though it is much more difficult to make good wine without sulfites. Vodka is actually less toxic than whiskey. If you doubt this, drink vodka on one night and then drink the same amount of whiskey on another night and compare how you feel in the morning. The "best" forms of alcohol are beer and wine.

Don't drink too much alcohol: keep it around 1 ounce per day for women and 2 ounces for men.

Use the Least Toxic Forms of Marijuana

If you use marijuana, use the forms that are least toxic. It's better to get forms of the herb that are organically grown to ensure that you are not inhaling toxic chemicals used in their cultivation. There is no more efficient way of getting these very toxic chemicals into your body than smoking them! Indoor growers will also tend to use a lot of pesticides and herbicides. If you use extracts, choose those extracted with carbon dioxide, since this means there will be no solvent residues.

To help you get started on the Toxin Solution Maintenance Plan here are fourteen days' worth of meal plans that follow the food guidelines in this chapter.

Table 8.3. **Meal Plans** (You can find more recipes at www.thetoxinsolution.com)

DAY 1	
Breakfast	Zucchini omelet with gluten-free toast
Midmorning snack	Coconut yogurt with chopped almonds and berries
Lunch	Turkey chili with GMO-free cornbread
Midafternoon snack	Oven-baked organic kale chips with avocado dip
Dinner	Garlic broccoli with lamb chop and dairy-free Caesar salad
DAY 2	
Breakfast	Scrambled eggs with rye crisp
Midmorning snack	Organic strawberry smoothie with hemp milk
Lunch	Watercress and sunflower seed salad with sardines, organic kale chips
Midafternoon snack	Avocado half with lemon
Dinner	Organic baked chicken, sweet potato, steamed broccoli, and green beans
DAY 3	
Breakfast	Gluten-free granola with yogurt and blueberries
Midmorning snack	Organic apple with almond butter
Lunch	Apple-celery-pecan chicken salad over greens with lemon-oil dressing
Midafternoon snack	Vegetable crudité with hummus
Dinner	Lamb moussaka with Greek salad
DAY 4	
Breakfast	Oatmeal with organic apples
Midmorning snack	Almond butter with sliced cucumber
Lunch	Turkey burger with lemony slaw
Midafternoon snack	Carrots with chickpea dip
Dinner	Stuffed cabbage with rice pilaf
DAY 5	
Breakfast	Deviled eggs with sesame green salad
Midmorning snack	Blueberry hemp shake
Lunch	Green goddess salad with chopped chicken, watercress, and sliced tomatoes
Midafternoon snack	Lentil chips with yogurt dill dip
Dinner	Braised wild-caught salmon, curried cauliflower, and green bean sauté with dilled cucumber salad

DAY 6	
Breakfast	Huevos rancheros with tortilla
Midmorning snack	Walnuts and pear
Lunch	Grilled vegetables with cauliflower "rice" and chopped salad
Midafternoon snack	Celery with sunflower-pecan spread
Dinner	Brassica stir-fry with wild salmon cakes
DAY 7	
Breakfast	Quinoa cereal with fresh fruit and dairy-free milk
Midmorning snack	Mocha hemp smoothie
Lunch	Lentil burgers with sesame green beans and napa cabbage salad
Midafternoon snack	Orange slices
Dinner	Gluten-free quinoa spaghetti and grass-fed bison meatballs with tomato-zucchini oreganata and tossed salad
DAY 8	
Breakfast	Hot amaranth cereal with toasted sesame seeds and hemp milk
Midmorning snack	Deviled eggs with sliced pepper
Lunch	Black beans with mushroom gravy in baked sweet-potato skins
Midafternoon snack	Baked apple
Dinner	Roast turkey breast with braised Brussels sprouts, kasha, and cranberry-orange sauce
DAY 9	
Breakfast	French toast topped with berries
Midmorning snack	Crudités with garlic-nut dip
Lunch	Cold red-beet borscht and turkey roll-up
Midafternoon snack	Green drink with whey protein
Dinner	Bison steak with broccoli and amaranth
DAY 10	
Breakfast	Cinnamon organic apple-nut porridge
Midmorning snack	Scoop of parsley/egg salad with chopped cucumber and tomato
Lunch	Turkey loaf with spinach-stuffed acorn squash
Midafternoon snack	Celery with garlic dip
Dinner	Chicken wings with sautéed garlic, broccoli, and corn on the cob

DAY 11	
Breakfast	Organic spinach-mushroom frittata
Midmorning snack	Chicken wings with crudités and creamy dressing
Lunch	Vegetable-and-bean chili topped with sprouts
Midafternoon snack	Berry cobbler with almond cream
Dinner	Nut-stuffed sweet potatoes, green beans, and red-cabbage slaw
DAY 12	
Breakfast	High-fiber cereal with berries
Midmorning snack	Walnuts with sliced organic apple
Lunch	Cheddar broccoli soup with turkey bacon and toasted sunflower seeds
Midafternoon snack	Guacamole with GMO-free chips
Dinner	Gluten-free pizza with chopped broccoli, garlic, and basil–pine nut pesto topping and Caesar salad
DAY 13	
Breakfast	Waffles with turkey bacon
Midmorning snack	Lentil salad with hard-boiled egg
Lunch	Bun-less burger with sliced tomato, avocado, and sauerkraut
Midafternoon snack	Wheat-free pita triangles with hummus
Dinner	Chinese chicken and green bean stir-fry over cauliflower rice
DAY 14	
Breakfast	Peach hemp smoothie and eggs over easy with gluten-free toast
Midmorning snack	Rainbow fruit salad
Lunch	Adzuki bean burger with stir-fried shiitake mushrooms and sprout salad
Midafternoon snack	Organic popcorn with olive oil and nutritional yeast
Dinner	Curried lamb over rice with dal and yogurt cucumber salad

Air

Unless you plan to move to an area with especially clean air, you are stuck with air pollution, especially when living in cities, and especially in those cities with smog. Even rural areas may have many local sources of pollution—from burning fossil fuels, air currents bringing pollution from elsewhere, rural industries, and even from your home's heating system. Fortunately, a number of strategies will greatly decrease your exposure to toxins in the air, wherever you encounter them.

First, you can filter the air you breathe in your house. Put HEPA (high-efficiency particulate arresting) filters in your bedrooms, family room, kitchen, and wherever else in your house you spend a lot of time. If your house uses forced-air heating or cooling, follow these specific guidelines:

- Have your furnace inspected annually to ensure there are no gas or oil leaks.

- Install the best-quality air filters you can afford, and change them regularly.

- Install electronic electrostatic filters, and clean them regularly.

I recommend that you *not* use an ozone machine to improve the air in your home or office. While the ozone is great at precipitating out the particles in the air, we are already exposed to way too much of this highly oxidative compound in city air. And avoid using air fresheners. According to the Natural Resources Defense Council (NRDC), rather than "freshening" your air, all they really do is release phthalates, volatile organic compounds (VOCs), and benzene and formaldehyde (both of which are carcinogens) into your home.[1] Same problem with the softeners put in driers. If you must use them, choose those without fragrance.

No matter how cozy or picturesque or off the grid it seems, another source of pollution is a wood-burning fireplace. Use an electric or gas fireplace instead, which will have fewer emissions. If you really want to get off the grid, try to hook up with a renewable energy source like solar or wind. If you're intent on the coziness of a wood fire, be very sure circulation is good and there are no leaks in the fireplace or flue.

Water

The water you get from your local water supply may be anywhere from relatively pure to very contaminated. You can ask your water supplier to provide you with a copy of the periodic assays required by the federal government. Alternatively, you can test the actual water you are drinking at home. I list in appendix G laboratories that test water for metal and chemical contamination. This is a real problem, since around 10 percent of public water supplies have elevated levels of arsenic. Water from wells in farming communities can also have high levels of nitrates, herbicides, and pesticides.

Chlorine, which is added to all water supplies to kill off pathogenic bacteria and parasites, conveys a huge public health benefit, since a lot of people, especially infants, were killed in the past by infections from polluted water. Those infecting organisms are killed by chlorine binding to their hydrocarbons and producing toxic chemicals that kill the bugs. On the other hand, the organic trihalomethane by-products of chlorination (chloroform, bromodichloromethane, chlorodibromomethane, and bromoform) are carcinogenic.[2] I read a paper years ago that reported that one out of every ten thousand people who are saved from infection gets cancer from these molecules. It's a very good public health trade-off—unless you are that one in ten thousand.

To ensure that your water is of very good quality, install a whole-house carbon block filter. This will give you pure water for cooking and also bathing. Most people don't realize that we absorb a lot more potentially carcinogenic hydrocarbons from breathing in a shower than from water when we drink it. If you can't put in a whole-house filter, put a carbon block filter on your shower and in the kitchen sink for your food.

Carbon Monoxide and Smoke Alarms

Most cities and states now require that all households have carbon monoxide and smoke alarms. Use them; they can save your life. There are two types of smoke alarms—photoelectric and ionization. Always choose the photoelectric kind. The ionization type of smoke alarm contains a small amount of radioactive material called americium-241. Test the batteries to make sure these are in working order. (If the smoke alarms are wired into your home's electricity, make sure the backup batteries are working.)

Natural Cleansers

I recommend using only cleaning products that are low in solvents, fragrances, and other chemicals. According to a list compiled by the natural products website GAIAM (www.experiencelife.com), common household cleaners harbor many substances harmful to human health. Here are some of the ingredients you should avoid:

- Chlorinated phenols (in toilet-bowl cleaners)

- Diethylene glycol (in window cleaners)

- Phenols (in disinfectants)

- Nonylphenol ethoxylate (in laundry detergents and all-purpose cleaners)

- Petroleum solvents (in floor cleaners)[3]

Unfortunately, you won't always find a complete ingredient list on product labels due to laws protecting trade secrets. That's one among many reasons that in our house my wife, Lara, and I use a special cleaning solution we call Lara's Solution that she makes from the following ingredients:

- Water (1 quart)

- White vinegar (2 to 3 ounces)

- Essential oils, typically lavender combined with rosemary or rose oil (8 to 10 drops)

To help keep the house clean and free of toxins, remove your shoes upon entering. The dirt and dust outside are often full of toxins precipitated from the air. For example, if you have a wooden deck or play sets for children, they constantly leak small amounts of preservatives with highly toxic arsenic or cadmium. Provide socks or washable slippers for guests. Vacuum and wipe surfaces regularly, particularly if you live in a city where there may be a lot of particulate matter and soot.

You will find my recommendations for safe cleaning products in appendix F.

Furnishings

Do not spray your furniture with "stain resistant" chemicals, which are highly toxic perfluorinated compounds. Instead, if furniture stains are a problem, buy nonfabric, nonplastic furniture—for example, leather, 100 percent organic cotton, cotton and linen blends, and wood. Or use coverings that are easily washable.

Bedding, especially "temperature sensitive" mattresses, can release a lot of VOCs directly into your breathing space for hours every night. Use bedding made from natural materials processed with minimal chemicals.

Mold

Check all areas of your house for black mold. This is a huge problem that occurs in as many as 50 percent of commercial and residential buildings. The chemicals and spores released by this mold disrupt the immune system and increase inflammation. I was quite surprised to learn that an amazing two-thirds of adult-onset asthma appears to be due to mold exposure. Although this occurs mostly in bathrooms and kitchens, where there is water, you should carefully check the outside of your house as well for leaks that may allow water into the insulation in the walls—a perfect incubating place for black mold. If you have a mold problem, I strongly recommend seeking the assistance of an expert, since what you see may be only the tip of a serious toxic iceberg damaging your health.

Clothing

Wear clothing made primarily from natural fibers—cotton, wool, hemp, or silk. Limit your wearing of "breathable" rain clothing, which usually contains perfluorochemicals. If you really want to use such types of clothing (and I admit that it's convenient; my motorcycle jacket and pants use treated fabric), don't try to renew them by spraying them when they wear out. Buy a new outfit.

For your children, use only clothing without polybrominated diphenyl ethers (PBDEs). Yes, this means that the clothes will be less resistant to fire, so be more careful. Your children are much more likely to be damaged by PBDEs than by fire.

House Paints

That fresh-paint smell we may love is caused by volatile organic compounds (VOCs), chemicals that evaporate at room temperature. These toxic chemicals, found with pigments, are also added to alkyd oil and some latex paints to provide spreadability and durability. Low-level exposure to these chemicals can cause headaches, dizziness, and nausea. Higher exposure and longer exposure times—like those experienced by people who work in paint spray booths—can cause permanent damage to the kidneys, liver, and nervous or respiratory system.

Many companies now make low- and no-VOC paints that work as well as their predecessors. But don't confuse low-odor with low-VOC. Some paints mask the odor while having high levels of VOC. Look for levels of 100 grams per liter (g/L) or lower. Paints also routinely contain solvents and other additives, like formaldehyde, that you don't want to inhale. Your best option is to use natural, earth-based paints and pigments if you can find them and are willing to put up with a slightly less "polished" look.

Interestingly, a study I just read summarized research showing that much of the mold toxicity is due to the VOCs that molds release when growing on building materials.

Health and Beauty

To keep reducing your toxic load, use only health and beauty aids (HABAs) that are low in chemicals. To know which these are, read the labels—and look at appendix F of this book. If a product you are using (for almost anything) has a nice fragrance, most likely it contains phthalates. The smell may be pleasant, but phthalates—used in hundreds of products as plasticizers or in solvents—are carcinogenic and known to cause reproductive damage. And as you can see in appendix C, they are one of the major causes of the diabetes epidemic. (See page 47 for more on phthalates.)

Continue Getting Out the Old Toxins

Obviously, you can't get out all the toxins you've spent years accumulating in just a few weeks. Yes, following the Toxin Solution will greatly lessen the load of toxins in your blood, cells, and intracellular spaces, but they will keep refilling from bone and fat until these sources are detoxed as well. This is not meant to discourage you. Instead, what I want to leave you with is the good news that you *can* continue to deepen your detox and improve your health over time. Remember the efforts that Jennifer, who had elevated lead and mercury levels, made in chapter 1? As her levels decreased, her health gradually and continually improved.

To continue getting out the old toxins, take the following actions:

- Implement as much of the above as you can. If you do nothing other than live as cleanly as possible, your body will continue to detoxify—albeit slowly. Again, the best strategy is to keep the toxins out.

- Continue eating cabbage-family foods. They are the best for supporting liver detoxification.

- Continue taking fiber supplements. If this is all you do, having fiber in your gut to absorb the toxins being excreted by your liver will greatly help your most important detoxification processes.

- Add a nourishing drink of blended green vegetables to your diet.

- Incorporate an occasional massage into your health regimen.

- Do something every week that gets you freely sweating for at least an hour. For me, it's playing basketball. For others, it's a sauna, a bike ride, or the treadmill. Lara likes Zumba and barre.

This chapter put you on the path to maintaining all of the gains you made on the Toxin Solution. By first following the recommended program for detoxing and then adopting the healthy habits I have recommended here, you can ensure that your body:

- Avoids toxins as much as possible.

- Eliminates toxins efficiently.

- Repairs any damage done by toxic overload.

By understanding these processes of toxification and detoxification, you have become your body's best friend, able to support your health for years to come.

Detoxifying and keeping toxins out are your most effective strategies for avoiding disease and extending your healthy years as far into the future as possible.

Thank you for taking this ride with me.

Appendices Introduction

The eight appendices in this section will help you:

- Determine your toxic load.
- Discover which toxins are your biggest problem.
- Provide resources to effectively help you avoid toxins in the future.

This information is not meant to be comprehensive. Rather, it consists of my recommendations based on products, services, and lab tests whose purity and accuracy I have tested wherever possible. They are also products that my family and I use ourselves. Apart from any already mentioned, I have no commercial interests in any of the products or companies listed.

I invite those wanting my most current recommendations to visit this book's website, www.thetoxinsolution.com, which describes many more free resources, along with tools for interpreting laboratory tests and genomics. The latter is particularly useful, because knowing your genetic susceptibilities will help you determine which toxins are most toxic for you.

A brief description of the purpose of each appendix follows.

Assessment Appendices

Appendix A: Conventional Lab Tests Indicating Toxic Load.
Directly and accurately measuring the levels of specific toxins in our
body is recommended. However, such tests are in the early stage of development, not readily available, and very costly. Ironically, we have another
way of objectively determining overall body load of toxins: we have
become so toxic that many conventional laboratory tests show variations
within the supposed "normal" range. The "normal" range now shows
toxin exposure. That's right, toxic is now "normal," which helps explain
why we have such a huge disease burden. These tests are very useful, since
they are inexpensive and can be run by any doctor or lab.

Unfortunately, since most of us are affected by several different toxins, these conventional lab tests will not tell us precisely which toxins
we are being exposed to. By using the simple assessment formula that I
provide, you can estimate how loaded your body is with toxins and can
track improvement over time.

Appendix B: Lab Tests for Specific Toxins. A growing number of laboratories have started to provide tests that assess body load of specific
toxins. These are still to some degree controversial. Nonetheless, I have
found them very helpful for a lot of patients not only to pinpoint exactly
which toxins are causing them trouble, but also to then track efficacy
of avoidance and elimination strategies. Most of these tests require the
assistance of a doctor knowledgeable in environmental medicine.

Appendix C: Diseases That Indicate Specific Toxins. Along with
my team, I have done a lot of work determining the specific toxins that
cause chronic disease. For over a year, the three of us delved deeply into
the research assessing the contribution to eighteen cancers and thirty
chronic diseases of twenty-six toxins or toxin classes (e.g., lead is a single
toxin, whereas the hundreds of chemicals categorized as PCBs are considered one toxin class). For many of the toxins we looked at, there was

insufficient research, or the studies were too small. But for about one-third of them with reliable data, the results are uniformly disconcerting. Most show strong disease relationships, with the strongest summarized here. Comparing the disease(s) you or your family are suffering with the toxins can quickly tell you which toxins are the worst for you.

Appendix D: Symptoms That Indicate Specific Toxins. While all the other assessment appendices are based on strong research, this one is much more dependent upon my subjective judgment. Frustratingly, almost all the research on symptoms caused by specific toxins is based on acute poisoning or chronic industrial exposure at moderate dosages. Obviously, it's better to recognize that we have a problem with a toxin long before it progresses to outright disease. This appendix will help you determine whether your symptoms are those typically caused by specific toxins.

Appendix E: Symptom Tracking. One of the challenges with natural therapies is that it takes time for the body to heal—as opposed to the quick symptom relief of drugs, which usually don't treat the cause and add to toxic load. I have seen that patients are typically focused on their current symptoms and forget those that have gone away as their body heals. Having them use a weekly questionnaire that can numerically track their progress over time—such as the one in this appendix—powerfully reinforces the benefits of making the effort to live healthfully. At my website I provide some really helpful tools for objectively tracking your health status.

Resource Appendices

Appendix F: Safe Products. This appendix lists resources for determining the safest foods, health and beauty aids, yard chemicals, and house-cleaning products. These are the resources my family and I use.

Again, this is not a comprehensive list, and I apologize to any company making safe products that has been left out. (If your product has been omitted and you think it should be listed here, please contact me and we will make an assessment and, if appropriate, put you on the website.)

Appendix G: Other Resources. If you have a high level of a specific toxin and want to determine where it is coming from, or just want to make your home and workplace as free of toxins as possible, these resources will help.

Appendix H: Protocol Summary. The protocol summary appendix provides an easy-to-use review of the key elements for each protocol stage.

Appendix A:
Conventional Lab Tests
Indicating Toxic Load

This appendix recommends conventional laboratory tests to help determine whether you are overloaded with toxins. The tests are listed alphabetically, not in order of importance.

Although these tests are typically used to detect disease and are not intended to assess toxicity, the research shows that within the supposed "normal" range they can indicate physiological adaptations to or damage from toxins. While the tests won't tell us the exact toxin or toxins that are causing the problem, they do suggest types of toxins. Their huge value is that they are inexpensive and easily available. Finally, there is a simple scoring method to help you determine your general level of toxicity. As an example, my total score is 6.0. My family and I do everything we can to decrease our toxic exposure. Nonetheless, doing this assessment myself alerts me that I need to do a bit better.

"Normal" ranges can vary to some degree by laboratory. If your lab test range is different, then rescale the results proportionately. For example, if the top of the range in your lab is 10 percent higher, then scale the toxic ranges by 10 percent.

Some tests also vary according to a person's nutritional status; for example, homocysteine levels are higher when people are deficient in B vitamins. Of particular importance, being high in lead makes the elevation of homocysteine due to B-vitamin deficiency even worse.

The scoring method is based on my interpretation of the strength of the predictive value of the tests.

Interpreting Lab Test Results

TEST NAME	TYPICAL TOXINS	NORMAL RANGE	TOXIC RANGE	TOXIC SCORE	YOUR SCORE
ALT (Alanine aminotransferase)	Cadmium, lead, mercury, OCPs, PCBs	0–35 U/L	0–24	0	
			25–30	1	
			31–35	2	
AST (Aspartate aminotransferase)	OCPs	0–35 U/L	0–23	0	
			24–26	1	
			27–35	2	
Bilirubin (total)	PCBs, PFOA, PFOS	0.3–1.2 mg/dL	0.3–0.7	0	
			0.8–1.0	1	
			1.1–1.2	2	
LDL-cholesterol	PCBs	≤130 mg/dL	<110	0	
			110–130	1	
GGTP (Gamma-glutamyl transferase)	Most toxins	10–50 U/L	10–20	0	
			21–30	2	
			31–45	4	
			46–50	8	
HbA1c	Most POPs	4.0–8.5 percent	4.0–5.5	0	
			5.6–6.0	1	
			6.1–6.4	3	
			>6.4	5	
Homocysteine	Cadmium, lead	4–12 µmol/L	4.0–8.0	0	
			8.1–10.0	1	
			10.1–12.0	2	
Platelet count	Benzene, solvents	150–400	150–200	2	
			201–250	1	
			251–400	0	

TEST NAME	TYPICAL TOXINS	NORMAL RANGE	TOXIC RANGE	TOXIC SCORE	YOUR SCORE
T3 (total)	PCBs, PFOAs	0.7–1.5 ng/dL	0.7–0.8	2	
			0.9–1.0	1	
			1.1–1.5	0	
T4 (total)	PCBs	4.9–11.7 ng/dL	4.9–5.9	2	
			6.0–7.9	1	
			8.0–11.7	0	
Uric acid (blood)	PFOA, PFOS	2.5–8.0 mg/dL	2.5–5.3	0	
			5.4–5.6	1	
			5.7–5.8	3	
			>5.8	5	
WBC (White blood cell count)	Benzene, CO, OCPs, PCBs	4,000–10,000	4,000–5,000	3	
			5,001–6,000	2	
			6,001–7,000	1	
			7,001–10,000	0	
YOUR TOTAL TOXIC SCORE					

How to Score Your Answers:

Low toxin load: < 5.0

Marginally toxic: 5.1–10.0

Modestly toxic: 10.1–15.0

Highly toxic: > 15.0

References for Appendix A

Gleason, J. A., G. B. Post, and J. A. Fagliano. "Associations of perfluorinated chemical serum concentrations and biomarkers of liver function and uric acid in the US population (NHANES), 2007–2010." *Environmental Research* 136 (2015): 8–14.

Guallar, E., E. K. Silbergeld, A. Navas-Acien, et al. "Confounding of the relation between homocysteine and peripheral arterial disease by lead, cadmium, and renal function." *American Journal of Epidemiology* 163, no. 8 (2006): 700–708.

Kumar, J., L. Lind, S. Salihovic, B. van Bavel, E. Ingelsson, and P. M. Lind. "Persistent organic pollutants and liver dysfunction biomarkers in a population-based human sample of men and women." *Environmental Research* 134 (2014): 251–56.

Lee, D. H., M. H. Ha, J. H. Kim, et al. "Gamma-glutamyltransferase and diabetes: A 4 year follow-up study." *Diabetologia* 46 (2003): 359–64.

Penell, J., L. Lind, S. Salihovic, B. van Bavel, and P. M. Lind. "Persistent organic pollutants are related to change in circulating lipid levels during a 5 year follow-up." *Environmental Research* 134 (2014): 190–97.

Serdar, B., W. G. LeBlanc, J. M. Norris, and L. M. Dickinson. "Potential effects of polychlorinated biphenyls (PCBs) and selected organochlorine pesticides (OCPs) on immune cells and blood biochemistry measures: A cross-sectional assessment of the NHANES 2003–2004 data." *Environmental Health* 13 (2014): 114.

Shih, H. T., C. L. Yu, M. T. Wu, et al. "Subclinical abnormalities in workers with continuous low-level toluene exposure." *Toxicology and Industrial Health* 27, no. 8 (2011): 691–99.

Shimizu, R., M. Yamaguchi, N. Uramaru, et al. "Structure-activity relationships of 44 halogenated compounds for iodotyrosine deiodinase-inhibitory activity." *Toxicology* 314, no. 1 (2013): 22–29.

Shrestha S., M. S. Bloom, R. Yucel, et al. "Perfluoroalkyl substances and thyroid function in older adults." *Environment International* 75 (2015): 206–14.

Steenland, K., S. Tinker, A. Shankar, and A. Ducatman. "Association of perfluorooctanoic acid (PFOA) and perfluorooctane sulfonate (PFOS) with uric acid among adults with elevated community exposure to PFOA." *Environmental Health Perspectives* 118, no. 2 (2010): 229–33.

Suarez-Lopez. J. R., D. H. Lee, M. Porta, M. W. Steffes, and D. R. Jacobs Jr. "Persistent organic pollutants in young adults and changes in glucose related metabolism over a 23-year follow-up." *Environmental Research* 137 (2015): 485–94.

Appendix B:
Lab Tests for Specific Toxins

The number of laboratories offering testing for toxins is growing. The following are laboratories that I have some experience with and am willing to recommend. For a more complete list and additional information, please go to www.thetoxinsolution.com.

LABORATORY	TESTS FOR	CONTACT	NOTES
Doctor's Data	Gut, metals	www.doctorsdata.com	Excellent for toxic metals
Genova Diagnostics	Gut, metals, POPs, solvents	www.gdx.net	Excellent for gut microbial balance
Quicksilver Scientific	Metals	www.quicksilverscientific.com	Experts in mercury
Great Plains Laboratory	Gut, POPs, solvents	www.greatplainslaboratory.com	Comprehensive chemical screen
Rocky Mountain Analytical	Solvents	www.rmalab.com	Basic toxin screen
US Biotek	Solvents	www.usbiotek.com	Basic toxin screen

To assess your body load of toxic metals, I strongly recommend the following assessment protocol, which must be done in collaboration with an environmental doctor. Basically, your first morning urine tells you current exposure, while the urine collected after you take the chelating agent assesses body load. This latter assessment is controversial, but it is the best one currently available without taking a biopsy. Please ask the environmental doctor whom you consult to assess whether or not there are any contraindications applicable to you in undertaking this protocol.

Assessment Protocol Instructions

Sample 1, for current exposure:

1. Collect first morning urine.
2. Send sample to lab.

Sample 2, for body load:

1. Take 300 mg of dimercaptopropane sulfonate (DMPS) and 500 mg of dimercaptosuccinic acid (DMSA). Access to these drugs requires a doctor.
2. Collect all your urine for the next six hours.
3. Send sample to lab.

Appendix C:
Diseases That Indicate
Specific Toxins

Although glyphosate is a common and serious toxin, as discussed in chapter 6, almost all the research has been done on the pure chemical rather than the far more toxic industrial product actually used. Therefore, it is not included here. You can see our latest compilation of the research, as well as all the references, at www.thetoxinsolution.com.

Blank cells mean that either we have not yet looked at the research, there is no research, or the available research is too limited or inconsistent. An *N* means the toxin does not appear to increase the risk of the disease. The number of asterisks shows the relative strength of the disease–toxin association and the apparent percentage of the disease due to the toxin.

Key Toxins by Disease

Blank = Research not yet reviewed, no available data, or insufficient or contradictory data
N = No apparent relationship
? = Theoretical mechanism, but not researched

Percentage of Disease Apparently Caused by Toxin
* = 3–5%
** = 6–10%
*** = 11–15%
**** = 16–40%
***** = >40%

	ADHD	ALS	Anxiety	Cancer, Bladder	Cancer, Breast	Cancer, Lung	Cancer, Lymphohematopoietic	Diabetes
Acrylamide	N				*		**	
Acrylonitrile						**		
Aluminum								
Arsenic				****		**	***	**
Benzene	N				**		**	
Bisphenol A		?	**					***
Cadmium	N					*		
Chloroform			N	*				
DDT	****	**			N	**	*	*
Dioxins							***	*
Fluoride					*			
Lead	**	**	N					
Mercury	**	**						
Organophosphate pesticides	**	**	**					
PCBs	****				**	*	?	***
Phthalates	**	?						****
Polybrominated diphenyl ethers	****							
Polycyclic aromatic hydrocarbons	****		***	**	**	***		****
Vinyl chloride		**				*		

Infertility	Juvenile IQ	Metabolic Syndrome	Myocardial Infarction	Obesity	Obstructive Lung Disease	Osteoporosis	Renal Disease	Thyroid Dysfunction	Blank = Research not yet reviewed, no available data, or insufficient or contradictory data N = No apparent relationship ? = Theoretical mechanism, but not researched **Percentage of Disease Apparently Caused by Toxin** * = 3–5% ** = 6–10% *** = 11–15% **** = 16–40% ***** = >40%
*									Acrylamide
*									Acrylonitrile
N	?					*			Aluminum
	***	**	*	N	N	*	*	**	Arsenic
*								N	Benzene
*		**	*	***	*			**	Bisphenol A
*	**		**		***	***	***		Cadmium
**									Chloroform
**				**	**				DDT
**		*		*					Dioxins
	****				*			*	Fluoride
**	***			?	**	*	*	N	Lead
**	*				*		*	**	Mercury
	*****								Organophosphate pesticides
*		**	****	**		N	*	***	PCBs
*		***							Phthalates
*					N				Polybrominated diphenyl ethers
*	***	***		***					Polycyclic aromatic hydrocarbons
*									Vinyl chloride

Appendix D:
Symptoms That Indicate
Specific Toxins

Like appendix C, "Diseases That Indicate Specific Toxins," the following table provides guidance on how your symptoms can indicate which toxins are damaging your body. The table is the result of my looking at a lot of research on chronic exposure.

Finding solid research on symptoms caused by various toxins is very difficult, since nearly all the research is on acute poisoning or chronic industrial exposure. There are very few controlled studies on the symptoms in the general population. That does not mean toxins don't produce symptoms. There is, however, a huge variation in each individual's toxin exposure, in a person's ability to get rid of toxins, and in his or her susceptibility to damage by specific toxins as well as by total toxic load.

The number of asterisks indicates the frequency with which a toxin causes a particular symptom. An effective way to use this table is to simply highlight your symptoms and see which toxins show up most frequently as potentially causing those symptoms. Combining these results with the toxins you may have found important in appendix C will be very helpful in prioritizing where you need to pay the most attention.

Symptoms by Toxins LEGEND * = Weak ** = Moderate *** = Strong **** = Very Strong	Anxiety	Brain fog	Depression	Dizziness	Drowsiness	Elevated blood pressure	Erectile dysfunction	Fatigue	Frequent infections	Headache	Insomnia
Acrylamide		**									
Acrylonitrile				*				**			
Aluminum	*	**	**								
Arsenic				*				*			
Benzene				**	**		*		*	**	
Bisphenol A						**	**		**		
Cadmium	*	**				**		**			
Chloroform		**						**	*	**	
DDT		**					*			**	
Dioxins		*						**		**	
Fluoride		*		*				*			
Lead	*	**	**			**	**	***		**	**
Mercury	**	**	**		**		**	***			**
Organochlorine pesticides		**					**		*		
Organophosphate pesticides	**	**				**		**		**	
PCBs		*						**	**		
Phthalates								**		**	
Polybrominated diphenyl ethers				**				**		**	
Polycyclic aromatic hydrocarbons									*	**	
Vinyl chloride				**	**			**		**	

Irritability	Joint pain	Loss of coordination	Loss of sense of touch	Memory loss	Metallic taste	Moodiness	Muscle weakness	Nausea	Nervousness	Rash on hands and feet	Tremor	
												LEGEND * = Weak ** = Moderate *** = Strong **** = Very Strong
		**	**			**						Acrylamide
**							**					Acrylonitrile
	**			*			**		*		*	Aluminum
		*	***					*		***		Arsenic
					*							Benzene
				**			*					Bisphenol A
	**	*		*	*				*		*	Cadmium
							***					Chloroform
**						*		**		*		DDT
**	**					*				*		Dioxins
		*						*				Fluoride
**		***	***	**	**	**	*		**		**	Lead
**		**		***	***	**			**		*	Mercury
						*		**	*	*	**	Organochlorine pesticides
				*		*	**	*	**	*	*	Organophosphate pesticides
	****	*		*			*	**				PCBs
		**					**					Phthalates
**												Polybrominated diphenyl ethers
						*		**				Polycyclic aromatic hydrocarbons
		**					**					Vinyl chloride

Appendix E:
Symptom Tracking

Medical Symptoms Questionnaire (MSQ)

Patient Name _____

Date _____

Rate each of the following symptoms based upon your typical health profile for the past 14 days. Track your score over time.

Point Scale   0 – *Never* or *almost never* have the symptom
1 – *Occasionally* have it; effect is *not severe*
2 – *Occasionally* have it; effect is *severe*
3 – *Frequently* have it; effect is *not severe*
4 – *Frequently* have it; effect is *severe*

`HEAD`

_____ Headaches
_____ Faintness
_____ Dizziness
_____ Insomnia   **TOTAL** _____

EYES

_____ Watery or itchy eyes

_____ Swollen, reddened or sticky eyelids

_____ Bags or dark circles under eyes

_____ Blurred or tunnel vision   **TOTAL** _____

(Does not include near- or far-sightedness)

EARS

_____ Itchy ears

_____ Earaches, ear infections

_____ Drainage from ear

_____ Ringing in ears, hearing loss   **TOTAL** _____

NOSE

_____ Stuffy nose

_____ Sinus problems

_____ Hay fever

_____ Sneezing attacks

_____ Excessive mucus formation   **TOTAL** _____

MOUTH/THROAT

_____ Chronic coughing

_____ Gagging, frequent need to clear throat

_____ Sore throat, hoarseness, loss of voice

_____ Swollen or discolored tongue, gums, lips

_____ Canker sores   **TOTAL** _____

SKIN

_____ Acne

_____ Hives, rashes, dry skin

_____ Hair loss

_____ Flushing, hot flashes

_____ Excessive sweating   **TOTAL** _____

HEART

_____ Irregular or skipped heartbeat
_____ Rapid or pounding heartbeat
_____ Chest pain   **TOTAL** _____

LUNGS

_____ Chest congestion
_____ Asthma, bronchitis
_____ Shortness of breath
_____ Difficulty breathing   **TOTAL** _____

DIGESTIVE TRACT

_____ Nausea, vomiting
_____ Diarrhea
_____ Constipation
_____ Bloated feeling
_____ Belching, passing gas
_____ Heartburn
_____ Intestinal/stomach pain   **TOTAL** _____

JOINTS/MUSCLES

_____ Pain or aches in joints
_____ Arthritis
_____ Stiffness or limitation of movement
_____ Pain or aches in muscles
_____ Feeling of weakness or tiredness   **TOTAL** _____

WEIGHT

_____ Binge eating/drinking
_____ Craving certain foods
_____ Excessive weight
_____ Compulsive eating
_____ Water retention
_____ Underweight   **TOTAL** _____

ENERGY/ACTIVITY

_____ Fatigue, sluggishness
_____ Apathy, lethargy
_____ Hyperactivity
_____ Restlessness   **TOTAL** _____

MIND

_____ Poor memory
_____ Confusion, poor comprehension
_____ Poor concentration
_____ Poor physical coordination
_____ Difficulty in making decisions
_____ Stuttering or stammering
_____ Slurred speech
_____ Learning disabilities   **TOTAL** _____

EMOTIONS

_____ Mood swings
_____ Anxiety, fear, nervousness
_____ Anger, irritability, aggressiveness
_____ Depression   **TOTAL** _____

OTHER

_____ Frequent illness
_____ Frequent or urgent urination
_____ Genital itch or discharge   **TOTAL** _____

                                           GRAND TOTAL _____

Used with permission from the Institute for Functional Medicine.

Appendix F:
Safe Products

Highest-Quality Nutritional and Herbal Supplements

Emerson Ecologics is a distributor of professional-grade nutritional supplements to the integrative health-care community. They independently assess quality standards of the manufacturers who want them to carry their products. You can find their assessments at: www.emersonecologics .com/Quality/QualitySummaries.aspx. I recommend buying products only from manufacturers rated Gold or better.

Safe Cosmetics

Campaign for Safe Cosmetics: www.safecosmetics.org

Safe Foods

Environmental Working Group: www.ewg.org

Safe Cleaning Products

The Honest Company: www.honest.com

Safe Cookware

Use stainless steel copper-bottomed cookware. A number of companies make such products.

Appendix G:
Other Resources

You can use the following resources to help you determine sources of toxins in your immediate world, decrease toxins in your home, and find doctors knowledgeable in environmental medicine. I have also included the names of those organizations whose conferences and trainings, in my opinion, provide doctors with the best education in this area. You can find many more good resources at www.thetoxinsolution.com. These are the ones my family uses.

Testing Water for Toxins

Metals. Doctor's Data: www.doctorsdata.com

Chemicals. Great Plains Laboratory: www.greatplainslaboratory.com

Determining Water and Air Toxins by Zip Code

Scorecard: www.scorecard.org

Decreasing Toxins in Water

LifeSource Water Systems: www.lifesourcewater.com (whole-house carbon block filter)

Doctors Knowledgeable in Environmental Medicine

Naturopathic doctors: www.naturopathic.org

Doctors who have completed the Functional Medicine fellowship
(this entails extensive training and a comprehensive examination for
competency): www.functionalmedicine.org

Doctors who have completed the Integrative Medicine fellowship
(this entails extensive training and a comprehensive examination for
competency): www.aihm.org

Best Conferences and Trainings for Doctors Interested in Environmental Medicine

American Association of Naturopathic Physicians annual conference:
www.naturopathic.org

Association for the Advancement of Restorative Medicine annual
conference: www.restorativemedicine.org

Academy of Integrative Health and Medicine annual conference and
training programs: www.aihm.org

Institute for Functional Medicine annual conference and training
programs: www.functionalmedicine.org

Genomic Testing

23andMe: www.23andme.com

Appendix H:
Protocol Summary

This sequence is carefully designed to safely take you through the process of decreasing toxin exposure, preparing your organs responsible for getting toxins out of your body and a final one-week intense protocol to help your cells release toxins so they can be eliminated.

Consult with your physician before beginning the protocol and do not begin the final week intensive detoxification before preparing your body to eliminate the toxins.

The following only include a few key elements from each protocol.

Weeks 1 and 2 (Chapter 3)

The purpose of these two weeks is to decrease your current exposure to toxins as much as possible.

Follow the diet on page 102.

- Only eat organically grown foods (if you can't afford these, only eat foods on the Clean15™ list).
- Do not eat any wheat, rye, or barley.

- Do not eat farmed fish.
- Eliminate alcohol and other recreational drugs.
- Eliminate salt and sugar.
- Eat plenty of cabbage-family foods.
- Use curcumin as a spice, not black pepper.
- Take a good-quality multistrain probiotic.
- Take a good-quality multivitamin and mineral supplement.
- Take a fiber supplement (not wheat bran).
- Drink plenty of pure, clean water.
- Only use health and beauty products without phthalates or other toxic chemicals.

Weeks 3 and 4 (Chapter 4)

This protocol helps clean up your gut, a major source of toxins for most people.

- Kill the bad bacteria in your gut with goldenseal root powder.
- Take fiber to bind the toxic chemicals released as the bad bacteria die.
- Reseed with good bacteria by taking a good-quality, multistrain probiotic.
- Repair your gut by drinking cabbage juice and taking the supplement quercetin and the herb licorice.

Weeks 5 and 6 (Chapter 5)

Preparing your liver, the major organ of detoxification, is critical for handling the toxins as they are released.

Follow the diet on pages 142 and 143.

- Take a good-quality B-vitamin complex supplement.
- Take the herbs dandelion and turmeric.
- Take NAC (N-acetyl cysteine).
- Take a fiber supplement.

- Apply topical glutathione.
- Avoid all forms of grapefruit.

Weeks 7 and 8 (Chapter 6)

Your kidneys are the second-most important detoxification and typically show the most damage over time from toxin exposure. Improving their function is critical for toxin elimination and long-term health.

Follow the diet on page 179.

- Carefully avoid all kidney-damaging agents like NSAIDs, salt, and phosphates.
- Take the herbs ginkgo biloba, ginger, and gotu kola.
- Take NAC (N-acetyl cysteine).
- Take mineral citrates.
- Drink beet juice twice a day.
- Drink plenty of clean water.
- Eat blueberries.

Week 9 (Chapter 7)

This protocol should not be implemented until the protocols preparing your organs of elimination have been completed. It is very important that you do not release toxins until your body is ready. During this week, which you can repeat as often as you want once your body is ready, you will intensely release toxins. If you become too uncomfortable, and certainly if you feel sick, please slow down the process by decreasing the length and frequency of saunas and eating more calories.

- Eat an alkalinizing diet (page 189).
- Consume 500 to 1,000 fewer calories a day.
- Drink green drinks.
- Take regular, long saunas while drinking extra water and taking electrolytes.
- Get a massage each week on the protocol.

Acknowledgments

Expressing appreciation to the special people who taught and collaborated with me is hazardous, as too many will be left unrecognized. Nonetheless, I must thank my teachers—Drs. John Bastyr, ND, DC; Sid Baker, MD; and Jeff Bland, PhD—and those who have walked the path with me: Sheila Quinn, who was so important to the creation of Bastyr University, and Michael Murray, ND, for the landmark *Textbook of Natural Medicine,* which showed the scientific basis of naturopathic medicine. Thank you, Gideon Weil, for your visionary understanding that led me to write the right book, and Alison Rose Levy, for your deep understanding of the toxicity problem and magically making my writing so much easier to understand. Also at HarperOne, I would like to thank Mark Tauber, Laina Adler, Terri Leonard, Lisa Zuniga, Nadea Mina, Julia Kent, Hilary Lawson, and Sydney Rogers. I also greatly appreciate the great guidance from my agents Celeste Fine and John Fine and partner Marc Isaacson, who made this book possible. Finally, special appreciation to Chrissie Cirovic, ND, and Geoff Bender, ND, for their great help reviewing the research.

Deepest appreciation to my loving and supportive family: wife Lara and children Raven and Galen.

References

Chapter 1

1. J. L. Carwile, X. Ye, X. Zhou, A. M. Calafat, and K. B. Michels, "Canned soup consumption and urinary bisphenol A: A randomized crossover trial," *Journal of the American Medical Association* 306, no. 20 (2011): 2218–20; S. Bae and Y. C. Hong, "Exposure to bisphenol A from drinking canned beverages increases blood pressure: Randomized crossover trial," *Hypertension* 65, no. 2 (2015): 313–19.

2. http://deainfo.nci.nih.gov/advisory/pcp/annualReports/pcp08–09rpt/PCP_Report_08–09_508.pdf.

3. http://www.sciencetimes.com/articles/6043/20150504/scientists-warn-chemicals-pizza-box.htm.

4. B. Mogensen, P. Grandjean, F. Nielsen, P. Weihe, and E. Budtz-Jørgensen, "Breastfeeding as an exposure pathway for perfluorinated alkylates," *Environmental Science and Technology* 49, no. 17 (2015): 10466–73. doi:10.1021/acs.est.5b02237.

5. http://www.sciencedaily.com/releases/2015/08/150820185905.htm.

6. https://www.goodreads.com/author/quotes/15332.Rachel_Carson.

7. http://www.nytimes.com/2010/05/06/opinion/06kristof.html?_r=0.

8. https://www.nlm.nih.gov/medlineplus/magazine/issues/summer11/articles/summer11pg6–8.html.

9. http://www.nytimes.com/2010/05/06/opinion/06kristof.html?_r=0.

10. http://ecowatch.com/2013/06/13/report-fracking-health-risks-pregnant
   -women-children/.

11. http://www.webmd.com/parenting/baby/news/20150603/fracking-linked-to
   -low-birth-weight-babies.

12. http://www.nrdc.org/water/drinking/qarsenic.asp.

13. http://www.theatlantic.com/health/archive/2014/03/the-toxins-that-threaten
   -our-brains/284466/.

14. http://pmep.cce.cornell.edu/profiles/extoxnet/TIB/manifestations.html.

15. http://pmep.cce.cornell.edu/profiles/extoxnet/metiram-propoxur/parathion-ext
   .html; http://pmep.cce.cornell.edu/profiles/extoxnet/TIB/manifestations.html.

16. L. Palkovicova, M. Ursinyova, V. Masanova, Z. Yu, and I. Hertz-Picciotto,
   "Maternal amalgam dental fillings as the source of mercury exposure in devel-
   oping fetus and newborn," *Journal of Exposure Science and Environmental
   Epidemiology* 18, no. 3 (2008): 326–31.

17. G. Guzzi, M. Grandi, C. Cattaneo, et al., "Dental amalgam and mercury levels
   in autopsy tissues: Food for thought," *American Journal of Forensic Medicine and
   Pathology* 27, no. 1 (March 2006): 42–45.

18. D. H. Lee, M. W. Steffes, A. Sjödin, R. S. Jones, L. L. Needham, and D. R.
   Jacobs Jr., "Low dose of some persistent organic pollutants predicts type 2 diabetes: A nested case-control study," *Environmental Health Perspectives* 118, no. 9
   (2010): 1235–42.

19. J. Fu, C. G. Woods, E. Yehuda-Shnaidman, et al., "Low-level arsenic impairs
   glucose-stimulated insulin secretion in pancreatic beta cells: Involvement of
   cellular adaptive response to oxidative stress," *Environmental Health Perspectives*
   118, no. 6 (2010): 864–70.

20. http://www.cdc.gov/tobacco/data_statistics/fact_sheets/adult_data/cig_smoking
   (accessed 8/16).

21. http://www.diabetes.org/advocacy/news-events/cost-of-diabetes.html.

22. K. M. Nelson, G. Reiber, and E. J. Boyko, "Diet and exercise among adults
   with type 2 diabetes: Findings from the Third National Health and Nutrition
   Examination Survey (NHANES III)," *Diabetes Care* 25, no. 10 (2002):
   1722–28.

23. S. Snitker, B. D. Mitchell, and A. R. Shuldiner, "Physical activity and prevention
   of type 2 diabetes," *Lancet* 361 (2003): 87–88.

24. W. Willett, J. Manson, and S. Liu, "Glycemic index, glycemic load, and risk of type 2 diabetes," *American Journal of Clinical Nutrition* 76 (2002): 274S–280S.

25. P. Wursch and F. X. Pi-Sunyer, "The role of viscous soluble fiber in the metabolic control of diabetes: A review with special emphasis on cereals rich in beta-glucan," *Diabetes Care* 20, no. 11 (1997): 1774–80.

26. J. Salmeron, F. B. Hu, J. E. Manson, et al., "Dietary fat intake and risk of type 2 diabetes in women," *American Journal of Clinical Nutrition* 73, no. 6 (2001): 1019–26.

27. M. D. Althuis, N. E. Jordan, E. A. Ludington, and J. T. Wittes, "Glucose and insulin responses to dietary chromium supplements: A meta-analysis," *American Journal of Clinical Nutrition* 76, no. 1 (2002): 148–55.

28. D. H. Lee, I. K. Lee, K. Song, et al., "A strong dose-response relation between serum concentrations of persistent organic pollutants and diabetes: Results from the National Health and Examination Survey 1999–2002," *Diabetes Care* 29, no. 7 (2006): 1638–44; D. H. Lee, I. K. Lee, M. Porta, M. Steffes, and D. R. Jacobs Jr., "Relationship between serum concentrations of persistent organic pollutants and the prevalence of metabolic syndrome among non-diabetic adults: Results from the National Health and Nutrition Examination Survey 1999–2002," *Diabetologia* 50, no. 9 (2007): 1841–51.

Chapter 2

1. http://www.healthandenvironment.org/partnership_calls/18271.

2. E. Konduracka, K. Krzemieniecki, and G. Gajos, "Relationship between everyday use cosmetics and female breast cancer," *Polskie archiwum medycyny wewnętrznej* 124, no. 5 (2014): 264–69.

3. http://time.com/4239561/johnson-and-johnson-toxic-ingredients/.

4. http://www.rodalewellness.com/health/cocamide-dea.

5. P. Factor-Litvak, B. Insel, A. M. Calafat, et al., "Persistent associations between maternal prenatal exposure to phthalates on child IQ at age 7 years," *PLoS One* 9, no. 12 (2014): e114003.

6. A. L. Ponsonby, C. Symeonides, P. Vuillermin, J. Mueller, P. D. Sly, and R. Saffery, "Epigenetic regulation of neurodevelopmental genes in response to in utero exposure to phthalate plastic chemicals: How can we delineate causal effects?" *Neurotoxicology* 55 (2016): 92–101. pii: S0161–813X(16)30089–4.

7. http://time.com/4239561/johnson-and-johnson-toxic-ingredients/; see also http://www.safecosmetics.org/get-the-facts/regulations/us-laws/lead-in -lipstick/.

8. http://cerch.org/research-programs/hermosastudy/.

9. S. E. Schober, L. B. Mirel, B. I. Graubard, et al., "Blood lead levels and death from all causes, cardiovascular disease, and cancer: Results from the NHANES III mortality study," *Environmental Health Perspectives* 114, no. 10 (2006): 1538–41.

10. S. Iqbal, P. Muntner, V. Batuman, and F. A. Rabito, "Estimated burden of blood lead levels 5 microg/dL in 1999–2002 and declines from 1988 to 1994," *Environmental Research* 107, no. 3 (2008): 305–11.

11. http://grist.org/politics/all-trump-ed-out-chris-christie-goes-home-to-block -funding-for-lead-poisoned-families/.

12. http://grist.org/politics/all-trump-ed-out-chris-christie-goes-home-to-block -funding-for-lead-poisoned-families/.

13. https://biologicaldiversity.salsalabs.com/o/2167/p/dia/action3/common/public /index.sjs?action_KEY=17435.

14. C. Bergkvist, M. Berglund, A. Glynn, A. Wolk, and A. Åkesson, "Dietary exposure to polychlorinated biphenyls and risk of myocardial infarction: A population-based prospective cohort study," *International Journal of Cardiology* 183 (2015): 242–48.

15. J. R. Suarez-Lopez, D. H. Lee, M. Porta, M. W. Steffes, and D. R. Jacobs Jr., "Persistent organic pollutants in young adults and changes in glucose related metabolism over a 23-year follow-up," *Environmental Research* 137 (2015): 485–94.

16. Suarez-Lopez et al., "Persistent organic pollutants."

Chapter 3

1. http://www.j-alz.com/press/2009/20090706.html.

2. http://www.huffingtonpost.com/2015/05/14/the-organic-effect_n_7244000 .html.

3. https://www.coop.se/PageFiles/430210/Coop%20Ekoeffekten_Rapport_eng .pdf.

4. http://ehp.niehs.nih.gov/120-a62/.

5. C. L. Curl, R. A. Fenske, and K. Elgethun, "Organophosphorus pesticide exposure of urban and suburban preschool children with organic and conventional diets," *Environmental Health Perspectives* 111 (2003): 377–82.

6. C. Gasnier, C. Dumont, N. Benachour, E. Clair, M. C. Chagnon, and G. E. Séralini, "Glyphosate-based herbicides are toxic and endocrine disruptors in human cell lines," *Toxicology* 262, no. 3 (2009): 184–91.

7. D. E. King, A. G. Mainous III, and C. A. Lambourne, "Trends in dietary fiber intake in the United States, 1999–2008," *Journal of the Academy of Nutrition and Dietetics* 112, no. 5 (2012): 642–48.

8. World Health Organization, "Dioxins and their effects on human health," Fact Sheet no. 225, http://www.who.int/mediacentre/factsheets/fs225/en/.

9. http://www.globalhealingcenter.com/nutrition/meat-and-dairy-toxins.

10. http://www.globalhealingcenter.com/nutrition/meat-and-dairy-toxins.

11. K. E. Nachman, P. A. Baron, G. Raber, K. A. Francesconi, A. Navas-Acien, and D. C. Love, "Roxarsone, inorganic arsenic, and other arsenic species in chicken: A U.S.-based market basket sample," *Environmental Health Perspectives* 121, no. 7 (2013): 818–24.

12. M. N. Jacobs, A. Covaci, and P. Schepens, "Investigation of selected persistent organic pollutants in farmed Atlantic salmon (Salmo salar), salmon aquaculture feed, and fish oil components of the feed," *Environmental Science & Technology* 36, no. 13 (2002): 2797–805.

13. http://www.seattletimes.com/seattle-news/environment/drugs-flooding-into -puget-sound-and-its-salmon/.

14. S. V. Adams, P. A. Newcomb, M. M. Shafer, et al., "Sources of cadmium exposure among healthy premenopausal women," *Science of the Total Environment* 409, no. 9 (2011): 1632–37.

15. http://wwf.panda.org/what_we_do/footprint/agriculture/soy/facts/.

16. http://www.nejm.org/doi/full/10.1056/NEJMp1505660?rss=mostEmailed&.

17. N. Benachour, H. Sipahutar, S. Moslemi, et al., "Time- and dose-dependent effects of Roundup on human embryonic and placental cells," *Archives of Environmental Contamination and Toxicology* 53, no. 1 (2007): 126–33.

18. G. E. Séralini, "Roundup toxicity and glyphosate-based herbicide toxicity," paper presented at the Environmental Medicine Conference, San Diego, March 2016; Benachour et al., "Time- and dose-dependent effects."

19. I. E. de Araujo, "Circuit organization of sugar reinforcement," *Physiology & Behavior* 164, pt. B (2016): 473–77. pii:S0031-9384(16)30189-5.

20. O. Levran, M. Randesi, J. C. da Rosa, et al., "Overlapping dopaminergic pathway genetic susceptibility to heroin and cocaine addictions in African Americans," *Annals of Human Genetics* 79, no. 3 (2015): 188–98.

21. X. Liu and K. Lv, "Cruciferous vegetables intake is inversely associated with risk of breast cancer: A meta-analysis," *Breast* 22, no. 3 (2013): 309–13.

Chapter 4

1. C. Cherbut, "Inulin and oligofructose in the dietary fibre concept," *British Journal of Nutrition* 87, suppl. 2 (2002): S159–62; J. A. Martínez, U. Etxeberría, A. Galar, and F. I. Milagro, "Role of dietary polyphenols and inflammatory processes on disease progression mediated by the gut microbiota," *Rejuvenation Research* 16, no. 5 (2013): 435–37.

2. D. A. De-Souza and L. J. Greene, "Intestinal permeability and systemic infections in critically ill patients: effect of glutamine," *Critical Care Medicine* 33, no. 5 (2005): 1125–35.

3. H. Kim, H. Kong, B. Choi, et al., "Metabolic and pharmacological properties of rutin, a dietary quercetin glycoside, for treatment of inflammatory bowel disease," *Pharmaceutical Research* 22, no. 9 (2005): 1499–1509.

4. D. Gupta, S. Agrawal, and J. P. Sharma, "Effect of preoperative licorice lozenges on incidence of postextubation cough and sore throat in smokers undergoing general anesthesia and endotracheal intubation," *Middle East Journal of Anesthesiology* 22, no. 2 (2013): 173–78.

5. W. D. Rees, J. Rhodes, J. E. Wright, L. F. Stamford, and A. Bennett, "Effect of deglycyrrhizinated liquorice on gastric mucosal damage by aspirin," *Scandinavian Journal of Gastroenterology* 14 (1979): 605–7.

6. N. Ebner, G. Földes, L. Schomburg, et al., "Lipopolysaccharide responsiveness is an independent predictor of death in patients with chronic heart failure," *Journal of Molecular and Cellular Cardiology* 87 (2015): 48–53.

7. M. I. Lassenius, K. H. Pietiläinen, K. Kaartinen, et al., "Bacterial endotoxin activity in human serum is associated with dyslipidemia, insulin resistance, obesity, and chronic inflammation," *Diabetes Care* 34, no. 8 (2011): 1809–15.

8. A. L. Neves, J. Coelho, L. Couto, A. Leite-Moreira, and R. Roncon-Albuquerque Jr., "Metabolic endotoxemia: A molecular link between obesity and cardiovascular risk," *Journal of Molecular Endocrinology* 51, no. 2 (2013): R51–64.

9. W. H. Tang, Z. Wang, B. S. Levison, et al., "Intestinal microbial metabolism of phosphatidylcholine and cardiovascular risk," *New England Journal of Medicine* 368, no. 17 (2013): 1575–84.

10. T. Suganami, K. Tanimoto-Koyama, J. Nishida, et al., "Role of the toll-like receptor 4/NF-kappaB pathway in saturated fatty acid–induced inflammatory changes in the interaction between adipocytes and macrophages," *Arteriosclerosis, Thrombosis, and Vascular Biology* 27 (2007): 84–91.

11. A. Everard and P. D. Cani, "Diabetes, obesity and gut microbiota," *Best Practice & Research Clinical Gastroenterology* 27, no. 1 (2013): 73–83; Neves et al., "Metabolic endotoxemia"; P. D. Cani, J. Amar, M. A. Iglesias, et al., "Metabolic endotoxemia initiates obesity and insulin resistance," *Diabetes* 56 (2007): 1761–72; Lassenius et al., "Bacterial endotoxin activity in human serum"; A. Alisi, M. Manco, R. Devito, et al., "Endotoxin and plasminogen activator inhibitor-1 serum levels associated with nonalcoholic steatohepatitis in children," *Journal of Pediatric Gastroenterology and Nutrition* 50, no. 6 (2010): 645–49.

12. C. Sostres, C. J. Gargallo, and A. Lanas, "Nonsteroidal anti-inflammatory drugs and upper and lower gastrointestinal mucosal damage," *Arthritis Research & Therapy* 15, suppl. 3 (2013): S3.

13. C. E. Ruhl and J. E. Everhart, "Fatty liver indices in the multiethnic United States National Health and Nutrition Examination Survey," *Alimentary Pharmacology & Therapeutics* 41, no. 1 (2015): 65–76.

14. Alisi et al., "Endotoxin and plasminogen activator inhibitor-1."

15. W. Nseir, F. Nassar, and N. Assy, "Soft drinks consumption and nonalcoholic fatty liver disease," *World Journal of Gastroenterology* 16, no. 21 (2010): 2579–88.

16. A. Spruss, G. Kanuri, S. Wagnerberger, S. Haub, S. C. Bischoff, and I. Bergheim, "Toll-like receptor 4 is involved in the development of fructose-induced hepatic steatosis in mice," *Hepatology* 50, no. 4 (2009): 1094–104.

Chapter 5

1. M. R. Fernandes, D. C. de Carvalho, Â. K. dos Santos, et al., "Association of slow acetylation profile of NAT2 with breast and gastric cancer risk in Brazil," *Anticancer Research* 33, no. 9 (2013): 3683–89.

2. G. Talska, H. Bartsch, N. Caporaso, et al., "Genetically based n-acetyltransferase metabolic polymorphism and low-level environmental exposure to carcinogens," *Nature* 369, no. 6476 (1994): 154–56.

3. A. Y. Leung, *Encyclopedia of Common Natural Ingredients Used in Food, Drugs and Cosmetics* (New York: John Wiley, 1980).

4. K. Faber, "The dandelion: *Taraxacum officinale* Weber," *Pharmazie* 13, no. 7 (1958): 423–36.

5. R. Kirchhoff, C. H. Beckers, G. M. Kirchhoff, H. Trinczek-Gärtner, O. Petrowicz, and H. J. Reimann, "Increase in choleresis by means of artichoke extract," *Phytomedicine* 1, no. 2 (1994): 107–15.

6. Y. Kiso, Y. Suzuki, N. Watanabe, Y. Oshima, and H. Hikino, "Antihepatotoxic principles of *Curcuma longa* rhizomes," *Planta Medica* 49, no. 3 (1983): 185–87.

7. T. M. Hagen, G. T. Wierzbicka, A. H. Sillua, B. B. Bowman, and D. P. Jones, "Bioavailability of dietary glutathione: Effect of plasma concentration," *American Journal of Physiology* 259, no. 4, pt. 1 (1990): G524–29.

8. J. Pangborn, *Mechanisms of Detoxification and Procedures for Detoxification* (West Chicago, IL: Bionostics, 1994), 115–18.

9. http://www.lifeextension.com/protocols/metabolic-health/metabolic -detoxification/Page-01.

10. R. J. Flanagan and T. J. Meridith, "Use of N-acetylcysteine in clinical toxicology," *American Journal of Medicine* 91, suppl. 3C (1991): 131S–139S; S. Kalghatgi, C. S. Spina, J. C. Costello, et al., "Bactericidal antibiotics induce mitochondrial dysfunction and oxidative damage in Mammalian cells," *Science Translational Medicine* 5, no. 192 (2013): 192ra85.

11. A. C. White, V. J. Thannickal, and B. L. Fanburg, "Glutathione deficiency in human disease," *Journal of Nutritional Biochemistry* 5, no. 5 (1994): 218–26; N. Ballatori, S. M. Krance, S. Notenboom, S. Shi, K. Tieu, and C. L. Hammond, "Glutathione dysregulation and the etiology and progression of human diseases," *Journal of Biological Chemistry* 390, no. 3 (2009): 191–214.

12. J. P. Richie Jr., "The role of glutathione in aging and cancer," *Experimental Gerontology* 27, nos. 5–6 (1992): 615–26.

13. http://www.atsdr.cdc.gov/substances/toxsubstance.asp?toxid=25.

14. J. A. Caruso, K. Zhang, N. J. Schroeck, B. McCoy, and S. P. McElmurry, "Petroleum coke in the urban environment: A review of potential health effects," *International Journal of Environmental Research and Public Health* 12, no. 6 (2015): 6218–31.

15. C. W. W. Beecher, "Cancer preventive properties of varieties of *Brassica oleracea*: A review," *American Journal of Clinical Nutrition* 59, no. 5, suppl. (1994): 1166S–70S.

16. P. L. Crowell and M. N. Gould, "Chemoprevention and therapy of cancer by d-limonene," *Critical Reviews in Oncogenesis* 5, no. 1 (1994): 1–22.

17. M. Nagabhushan and S. V. Bhide, "Curcumin as an inhibitor of cancer," *Journal of the American College of Nutrition* 11, no. 2 (1992): 192–98.

18. M. L. Pelchat, C. Bykowski, F. F. Duke, and D. R. Reed, "Excretion and perception of a characteristic odor in urine after asparagus ingestion: A psychophysical and genetic study," *Chemical Senses* 36, no. 1 (2011): 9–17.

19. J. E. Gallagher, R. B. Everson, J. Lewtas, M. George, and G. W. Lucier, "Comparison of DNA adduct levels in human placenta from polychlorinated biphenyl exposed women and smokers in which CYP 1A1 levels are similarly elevated," *Teratogenesis, Carcinogenesis, and Mutagenesis* 14, no. 4 (1994): 183–92.

20. H. J. Beijer and C. J. de Blaey, "Hospitalisations caused by adverse drug reactions (ADR): A meta-analysis of observational studies," *Pharmacy World & Science* 24, no. 2 (2002): 46–54.

21. J. Lazaraou, B. H. Pomeranz, and P. N. Corey, "Incidence of drug reactions in hospitalized patients: A meta-analysis of prospective studies," *Journal of the American Medical Association* 279, no. 15 (1998): 1200–1205.

22. P. Nourjah, S. R. Ahmad, C. Karwoski, and M. Willy, "Estimates of acetaminophen (Paracetamol)-associated overdoses in the United States," *Pharmacoepidemiology and Drug Safety* 15, no. 6 (2006): 398–405.

Chapter 6

1. http://www.atsdr.cdc.gov/substances/toxorganlisting.asp?sysid=20, accessed July 7, 2016.

2. C. J. White, "Catheter-based therapy for atherosclerotic renal artery stenosis," *Circulation* 113, no. 11 (2006): 1464–73.

3. L. Pizzorno, "Canaries in the phosphate-toxicity coal mines," *Integrative Medicine—A Clinician's Journal* 13, no. 6 (2014): 24–31.

4. M. Pruijm, L. Hofmann, J. Charollais-Thoenig, et al., "Effect of dark chocolate on renal tissue oxygenation as measured by BOLD-MRI in healthy volunteers," *Clinical Nephrology* 80, no. 3 (2013): 211–17.

5. A. L. Al-Malki and S. S. Moselhy, "The protective effect of epicatechin against oxidative stress and nephrotoxicity in rats induced by cyclosporine," *Human & Experimental Toxicology* 30, no. 2 (2011): 145–51.

6. S. M. Mansour, A. K. Bahgat, A. S. El-Khatib, and M. T. Khayyal, "Ginkgo biloba extract (EGb 761) normalizes hypertension in 2K, 1C hypertensive rats: Role of antioxidant mechanisms, ACE inhibiting activity and improvement of endothelial dysfunction," *Phytomedicine* 18, nos. 8–9 (2011): 641–47.

7. K. Cavuşoğlu, K. Yapar, E. Oruç, and E. Yalçin, "Protective effect of *Ginkgo biloba* L. leaf extract against glyphosate toxicity in Swiss albino mice," *Journal of Medicinal Food* 14, no. 10 (2011): 1263–72.

8. G. Sener, O. Sehirli, A. Tozan, A. Velioğlu-Ovunç, N. Gedik, and G. Z. Omurtag, "Ginkgo biloba extract protects against mercury(II)-induced oxidative tissue damage in rats," *Food and Chemical Toxicology* 45, no. 4 (2007): 543–50; K. Yapar, K. Cavuşoğlu, E. Oruç, and E. Yalçin, "Protective role of Ginkgo biloba against hepatotoxicity and nephrotoxicity in uranium-treated mice," *Journal of Medicinal Food* 13, no. 1 (2010): 179–88; A. Tozan, O. Sehirli, G. Z. Omurtag, S. Cetinel, N. Gedik, and G. Sener, "Ginkgo biloba extract reduces naphthalene-induced oxidative damage in mice," *Phytotherapy Research* 21, no. 1 (2007): 72–77.

9. F. C. Onwuka, O. Erhabor, M. U. Eteng, and I. B. Umoh, "Protective effects of ginger toward cadmium-induced testes and kidney lipid peroxidation and hematological impairment in albino rats," *Journal of Medicinal Food* 14, nos. 7–8 (2011): 817–21; A. A. Baiomy and A. A. Mansour, "Genetic and histopathological responses to cadmium toxicity in rabbit's kidney and liver: Protection by ginger (*Zingiber officinale*)," *Biological Trace Element Research* 170, no. 2 (2015): 320–29.

10. M. K. Kim, S. W. Chung, D. H. Kim, et al., "Modulation of age-related NF-kappaB activation by dietary zingerone via MAPK pathway," *Experimental Gerontology* 45, no. 6 (2010): 419–26.

11. K. R. Shanmugam, C. H. Ramakrishna, K. Mallikarjuna, and K. S. Reddy, "Protective effect of ginger against alcohol-induced renal damage and antioxidant enzymes in male albino rats," *Indian Journal of Experimental Biology* 48, no. 2 (2010): 143–49; A. A. Baiomy, H. F. Attia, M. M. Soliman, and O. Makrum, "Protective effect of ginger and zinc chloride mixture on the liver and kidney alterations induced by malathion toxicity," *International Journal of Immunopathology and Pharmacology* 28, no. 1 (2015): 122–28.

12. Z. Wang, J. Liu, and W. Sun, "Effects of asiaticoside on levels of podocyte cytoskeletal proteins and renal slit diaphragm proteins in adriamycin-induced rat nephropathy," *Life Sciences* 93, no. 8 (2013): 352–58.

13. X. M. Meng, Y. Zhang, X. R. Huang, et al., "Treatment of renal fibrosis by rebalancing TGF-β/Smad signaling with the combination of Asiatic acid and naringenin," *Oncotarget* 6, no. 35 (2015): 36984–97. doi:10.18632/oncotarget.6100.

Chapter 7

1. R. J. Colman, T. M. Beasley, J. W. Kemnitz, S. C. Johnson, R. Weindruch, and R. M. Anderson, "Caloric restriction reduces age-related and all-cause mortality in rhesus monkeys," *Nature Communications* 5 (2014): 3557.

2. M. E. Sears, K. J. Kerr, and R. I. Bray, "Arsenic, cadmium, lead, and mercury in sweat: A systematic review," *Journal of Environmental and Public Health* 2012:184745.

3. K. H. Kilburn, R. H. Warsaw, and M. G. Shields, "Neurobehavioral dysfunction in firemen exposed to polychlorinated biphenyls (PCBs): Possible improvement after detoxification," *Archives of Environmental Health* 44, no. 6 (1989): 345–50.

4. J. L. Stauber and T. M. Florence, "A comparative study of copper, lead, cadmium and zinc in human sweat and blood," *Science of the Total Environment* 74 (1988): 235–47.

5. A. Rodhe and A. Eriksson, "Sauna deaths in Sweden, 1992–2003," *American Journal of Forensic Medicine and Pathology* 29, no. 1 (2008): 27–31.

6. C. W. Nho and E. Jeffery, "The synergistic upregulation of phase II detoxification enzymes by glucosinolate breakdown products in cruciferous vegetables," *Toxicology and Applied Pharmacology* 174, no. 2 (2001): 146–52.

7. M. Basiri-Moghadam, K. Basiri-Moghadam, M. Kianmehr, and S. Jani, "The effect of massage on neonatal jaundice in stable preterm newborn infants: A randomized controlled trial," *Journal of Pakistan Medical Association* 65, no. 6 (2015): 602–6.

Chapter 8

1. http://www.nrdc.org/living/healthreports/hidden-hazards-air-fresheners.asp.

2. J. K. Dunnick and R. L. Melnick, "Assessment of the carcinogenic potential of chlorinated water: Experimental studies of chlorine, chloramine, and trihalomethanes," *Journal of the National Cancer Institute* 85, no. 10 (1993): 817–22.

3. http://experiencelife.com/article/8-hidden-toxins-whats-lurking-in-your -cleaning-products.

Index

Page references followed by *fig* indicate an illustrated figure; followed by *t* indicate a table.

acetaminophen (Tylenol): detoxification of, 169–70, 171*fig*; toxicity of, 86, 170

acrylates exposure, 46*t*

activated intermediate toxin, 164

ADHD (attention deficit hyperactivity disorder): lead levels increased with, 53*t*; pesticides toxicity and risk of, 31*t*, 88

adults: organophosphates and risk for dementia in elderly, 88*fig*; PCBs accumulation in, 61*fig*, 62–65; symptoms of lead exposure in, 52–53*t*

adverse drug reactions (ADRs), 168–69

age differences: adverse drug reactions (ADRs) and, 168; deterioration in kidney function and, 180*fig*; liver detoxification capacity and, 166; PCBs accumulation and, 61*fig*, 62–65; toxic exposures, health challenges by, 43*fig*

Agent Orange, 81

air pollution: benzene, 3–4, 26*t*, 213; mercury toxicity in, 26*t*; OCPs (organochlorine pesticides), 4; PAHs (polycyclic aromatic hydrocarbons), 31*t*; PBDEs (polybrominated diphenyl ethers), 4, 84*fig*; PCBs (polychlorinated biphenyls), 4, 26*t*, 31*t*, 35*fig*, 58, 59–65, 85, 86*fig*, 195*t*; PFASs (perfluorinated alkylated substances), 16–17, 195*t*; PFCs (perfluorinated chemicals), 4; POPs (persistent organic pollutants), 85, 101, 175, 178, 195*t*; strategies for avoiding, 212–13; VOCs (volatile organic compounds), 4, 213, 216, 217

alcohol: CYP2E1 (cytochrome P450 2E1) detoxification of, 132; as depleting body's glutathione stores, 95, 132–33, 150; general guidelines for safe consumption of, 133, 209; impact on gut and digestive tract by, 131, 132–34*fig*; understanding toxicity of, 95–96

Aleve, 86

alkaline diet, 189–90, 192

ALS (amyotrophic lateral sclerosis), 31*t*

aluminum exposure: aluminum cookware exposure to, 208; in health and beauty aids, 46*t*; synergistic effects of pesticides and, 30*fig*

Alzheimer's disease, 71, 143, 208. *See also* dementia

amalgams ("silver fillings") mercury toxicity, 25–26*t*, 27

American Medical Association (AMA), 14, 145

americium-214, 214

anemia: kidney damage and, 12*t*; as symptom of increased lead levels, 53*t*

anthocyanins, 185

antibiotics, 86

antifreeze (ethylene glycol), 175

aphthous stomatitis, 128

apples: Dirty Dozen food, 74; EU ban against American, 71; organic, 71–72

arsenic exposure: CDC on danger of, 84–85; detoxification through saunas, 195*t*; half-life in blood, 26*t*; hormone imbalance due to, 24–25; Portland's cadmium and, 56–58; specific disease risk associated with, 31*t*; synergistic effects of pesticides and, 30; water contamination, 18, 96; wooden decks and play sets that have, 215

artichoke extract, 142*t*, 152

artificial flavors, 11, 80–81

artificial sweeteners, 11, 81, 93, 205*t*, 206*t*. *See also* sugar

asparagus: asparagusic acid in, 167–68; Clean 15 food, 99

aspartame, 81

asthma: increasing rates of, 18; PAHs association with risk of, 31*t*; toxic exposures and, 43*t*, 128

atherosclerosis, 125

atopic dermatitis, 128

autism, 18

avocados, 99

bad bacteria. *See* gut bacteria

Baker, Sid, 79

Bastyr University, 122

Bastyr, John, 14

beef elimination, 84–85

beetroot juice, 186*fig*–87

benzene: caution against air fresheners that release, 213; daily exposure to, 3–4; DNA damage due to, 4; half-life in blood, 26*t*

benzofuran, 175

BHT toxicity, 80

Bifidobacterium species, 114*t*, 120

bile (liver), 147, 148

birth defects: prenatal mercury exposure and, 27; prenatal phthalates exposure and, 47–48*fig*

bisphenol A (BPA): increased toxic exposure to, 4–5, 80; levels by type of container, 5*fig*

black mold toxicity, 6, 216, 217

black pepper, 100

bladder cancer, 144

Blastocystis hominis, 128

blood: detox by kidneys during filtering of, 175–76, 179–81*fig*; half-lives of typical toxins in the, 26*t*; kidney detox capacity and impaired microcirculation of, 180; liver detox of the liver filtering the, 147, 148. *See also* hematological toxicity; microcirculation

blood-sugar levels: the heart, endotoxins, and, 127*fig*–28; impact of toxins on, 5; Noreen's story on detoxification and, 94*fig*; Two-Week Jumpstart Diet and people with variable, 105–6. *See also* Type 1 diabetes; Type 2 diabetes

blueberries, 179*t*, 186, 187

the body: capacity to heal by, 3; DNA of, 4, 5, 23, 24, 64, 80; eight ways toxins damage our, 23–25; genetic variability in liver susceptibility and detox of the, 29, 167–69; gluthathione stores protection from toxic damage to, 29; how chemical toxins dysregulate your, 22–23; intense full-body detox of, 191–99; interconnectivity of detoxification organs of, 173; knowing your personal detox capacity of, 144; preparing physically and psychologically for detox of, 138; Two-Week Diet and expected responses of your, 104–5. *See also* gut and digestive tract; kidneys; liver

Bone, Kerry, 184–85

bone loss, 7, 24, 90

BPA (bisphenol A), 208

brassica-family foods, 98–99, 164, 165

Breast Cancer Fund, 46

breast cancer risk, 31*t*, 40

breast-feeding: PFASs exposure through, 17; woman's chemical toxin load decreased with, 61–62*fig*

breathing protocol: alkalinizing your tissues with, 189–90; kidney detox instructions, 179*t*

bromodichloromethane, 175

bromoform, 175

B vitamins, 142*t*, 164, 165, 166–67, 178

cabbage: Clean 15 food, 99; healing the gut walls with, 120–21

cadmium toxicity: detoxification through saunas, 195*t*; fertilizers contaminated with, 207; half-life in blood, 26*t*; increasing rates of, 90; kidney detox of, 178; Portland's exposure of arsenic and, 56–58; soy products, 90–91; wooden decks and play sets that have, 215

caloric restriction: health benefits of, 193; healthy strategies for, 193; during intense full-body detox week, 192–93. *See also* fasting

Campaign for Safe Cosmetics (2007), 48, 49

cancer: artificial sweeteners linked to, 81; bladder, 144; breast, 31*t*, 40; how the liver's detox systems prevent, 143–44; increasing rates of, 13; links between water chlorination and incidence of, 214; lung, 31*t*; Peter's and Don's stories on, 15; specific toxins associated with risk of, 31*t*; Two-Week Jumpstart Diet and patients with, 105–6

Candida albicans, 128

cantaloupes, 99

carbon monoxide alarms, 204*t*, 214

cardiovascular heart disease: atherosclerosis and, 125; caution before using a sauna if you have, 197; endotoxins connected to, 123, 125, 126*fig*; increasing rates of, 12–13; metabolic endotoxemia (ME) and, 129; toxins related to, 40

Carroll, Robert, 114–15

Carson, Rachel, 13, 17

cauliflower, Clean 15 food, 99

cayenne pepper, 100

celery, 74, 88

celiac disease, 81, 128

cell membranes: how toxins damage, 24; "signaling" process of, 26

Center for Environmental Health (CEH), 46

Center for the Environment and Health, 18

Centers for Disease Control and Prevention (CDC): blood lead levels (BLLs) according to, 51; on toxicity of arsenic, 84–85

Charles's story, 182, 184–85

chemical toxicity: body dysregulation due to, 22–23; detoxification through saunas, 195*t*, 196; distinguishing between avoidable and unavoidable toxins, 39–40; food preservatives and additives, 205*t*–6*t*; health and beauty aids (HABAs), 6, 10, 11, 43, 45–49; Jack's story on, 19–21; liver enzymes work at breaking down, 100, 101, 147, 148–49, 155–56, 157–60; specifically targeting the kidneys, 174–75; Susan's story on, 146–47; Toxic Troubleshooter to assess your exposure to, 41–43, 171. *See also* detoxification; pesticides toxicity; *specific toxin*

chest pain, 174

chicken toxicity, 84–85

children: blood lead levels (BLLs) of, 51–52*fig*; childhood obesity rates in, 18; symptoms of increased lead levels in, 52–53*t*; toxicity and ADHD in, 31*t*, 53*t*, 88; Two-Week Jumpstart Diet medical supervision for, 105–6. *See also* infants

chlordane, 26*t*

chlordecone, 175

chlorination, 214

chlorobenzene, 175

chloroform, 175

chocolate, 186, 187

choline: conversion to TMA from, 125, 126*fig*; foods that produce, 165

Cipro, Darvon, 86

Clean 15 foods list: kidney detox and eating from, 189; as one of the Do's, 97; Sheryl's story on, 77; vegetables on the, 99–100 clean water, 189

clothing recommendations, 175, 216–17

coal tar derivatives, 175

coffee, 101

cognition: IQ levels and toxicity, 19, 53*t*, 78, 88*fig*; kidney damage and decreased, 174; memory loss, 53*t*; neurological toxicity symptoms, 12*t*; pesticides toxicity and U.S. elderly, 88*fig*. *See also* dementia

Collaborative on Health and the Environment, 45

conjugation process, 126

Connie's story, 54–55

Conrad's story, 109–12, 154

constipation, 53*t*

consumer-product toxins: clothing and furnishings, 175, 216–17; toxic overload due to, 12

conventional medicine. *See* health care

cooking technique recommendations, 208–9

COPD (chronic obstructive pulmonary disease), 197

Cornell University, 22

Crinnion, Walter, 13

CSA (community-supported agriculture), 203

cucumbers, 74

curcumin supplement, 142*t*, 179*t*, 186, 187

C vitamin, 142*t*, 165, 167

cysteine-rich foods, 165

cytochrome P450 2E1 (CYP2E1) enzyme, 132

dairy products: lactose intolerance to, 83, 84; as primary phosphate source, 183*t*

dandelion supplement, 142*t*, 152

Darvon, Cipro, 86

DDT: fish contaminated with, 85, 86*fig*; half-life in blood, 26*t*; risk of diseases associated with, 31*t*, 35*fig*

de la Monte, Suzanne, 71

dementia: alcoholism and, 133; toxicity and risk of, 78, 88*fig*; toxicity sometimes dismissed as, 8. *See also* Alzheimer's disease; cognition

depression: Ed's story on toxic foods and,

82–83; as leaky gut symptom, 113; Mildred's story on, 43–45; as symptom of toxicity, 12*t*; toxicity sometimes dismissed as, 8

dermatological toxicity: alcoholism and, 133; symptoms of, 12*t*

detoxification: of acetaminophen (Tylenol), 169–70; author's journey to practice of, 13–15; the body's reaction during, 151–54; Conrad's story on, 109–12, 154; fiber as critical to, 78–79, 101, 148; gut and digestive tract, 108–34; how toxins can impair your ability for, 25; importance to everyone's health, 36–37; interconnectivity of the body's organs of, 173; Jack's story on, 19–21; knowing your body's capacity for, 144; mercury- and lead-removal support of, 7–8; naturopathic medicine's focus on, 10, 11, 14–15, 64, 145; the practitioner's journey toward practicing, 9–11; reactions to, 151; Sally's story on, 72–74; Sheryl's story on, 76–78; strategies for maintaining, 210–19; three key determinants for health and successful, 9; Toxin Solution Maintenance Plan after successful, 202–19; water drinking recommendation during, 98, 179*fig*, 189. *See also* chemical toxicity; kidneys detoxification; liver detoxification; toxic load

detoxification diets: intense full-body detox (Week 9), 191–99; introduction to the Nine-Week Toxin Solution, 10, 49–50; learning and practicing detox protocols with, 10; mercury- and lead-removal support protocol combined with, 7–8; strategies for maintaining success of, 210–19; Toxin Solution Maintenance Plan after successful, 202–19; Two-Week Gut Protocol (Weeks 3 and 4), 109–14*t*, 117–22, 129–30, 135–36; Two-Week Jumpstart Diet (Weeks 1 and 2), 10, 45, 69–70, 74, 78–82, 97–106; Two-Week Kidney Detox Protocol (Weeks 7 and 8), 171–90; Two-Week Liver Detox Protocol (Weeks 5 and 6), 140–72. *See also* diet; food toxins detoxification strategies: actively promoting, 10; building detox capacity, 10; evading avoidable toxins, 9; repairing the damage, 10; repairing the detox organs, 9; your commitment to building capacity for, 9

Detox Maintenance Protocol: avoid additives and preservatives, 175, 203–4*t*; avoiding air and water pollution, 212–14; avoid teflon and aluminum cookware, 208; black mold checks, 216; carbon monoxide and smoke alarms, 204*t*, 214; clothing without toxins, 216–17; continue getting out the old toxins, 218–19; do not buy food packaged in plastic, 207–8; eat organically grown food, 203; furnishings without toxins, 216; grow some of your own food, 207; house paints without toxins, 217; limit alcohol consumption, 209; meal plans recommendations, 210*t*–12*t*; natural cleansers, 215–16; recommended cooking techniques, 208–9; reducing your use of toxic HABAs, 10, 43, 204*t*, 217–18; use the least toxic forms of marijuana, 209

DGL, deglycyrrhizinated licorice, 121–22

diabetes. *See* Type 1 diabetes; Type 2 diabetes

diarrhea, 12*t*

dibromoethane, 175

dibutyl phthalate (DBP) exposure, 46*t*, 47

dichloroethene, 175

dieldrin, 26*t*

diet: alkaline, 189–90, 192; kidney damage due to excessive phosphates in, 182; kidney damage due to excessive protein in, 182; low-protein, 166. *See also* detoxification diets

diethanolamine (DEA) exposure, 46*t*

diethyl phthalate exposure, 47

digestive problems. *See* leaky gut

dioxanes, 175

Dirty Dozen Plus Two list: description of the, 71; Detox Maintenance Protocol and avoidance of, 203; fruits and vegetables, 74; kidney detox and avoidance of, 189; worst vegetables included in the, 88

diseases: cancer, 15, 31*t*, 81, 106, 143–44;

cardiovascular disease, 12, 40, 123, 125, 126*fig*, 129, 197; caution regarding taking a sauna if you have serious, 197; *Encyclopedia of Natural Medicine* on treating, 132; failure of conventional medicine to address toxicity and, 21–22; gut toxins causing specific, 124–28; liver detoxification affecting all risks of, 140, 145; metabolic endotoxemia (ME) and associated, 128, 129–30; risk due to specific toxins, 31*t*–32; understanding how toxins cause, 1–2, 5–6, 23–25. *See also* Type 1 diabetes; Type 2 diabetes

DMDM hydantoin exposure, 46*t*

DNA: how benzene damages, 4; how toxins undermine repair and recovery of, 5, 24; polychlorinated biphenyls (PCBs) impact on, 64; as toxicity damage factor, 23, 80

Doctors Data, 96

Don's story, 15–16

D vitamin deficiency, 133

dyslipidemia, 129

E (IgE) blood tests, 82

Ed's story, 82–83

eggplant, 99

eggs: as primary phosphate source, 183*t*; as protein-rich food, 85, 182

EMFs exposure, 4

encephalopathy, 53*t*

Encyclopedia of Natural Medicine, 132

endocrine disruptors (EDCs): HERMOSA study on reducing, 50; phthalates as, 31*t*, 47–48*fig*

endotoxin metabolites: definition of, 112–13; how they disrupt the metabolism, 127*fig*; impact on the body by, 123–24, 133

energy: experiencing upsurge in weeks 7 and 8, 176; Sally's story on her lack of, 72–74; toxin interference with hormones causing lack of, 25

Enriching Blueberry Greens, 198

Entamoeba histolytica, 128

environmental toxins everyday exposures, 1–2, 5–6, 16–19

Environmental Working Group (EWG): Dirty Dozen food list of the, 71, 74, 88; Skin Deep database of the, 46

enzymes: cytochrome P450 2E1 (CYP2E1), 132; health as all about optimizing, 115–16; lactase, 83; liver-detoxification, 100, 101, 147, 148–49, 155–56, 157–60; nutrient deficiency impact on, 89*fig*–90; toxicity damage to, 23–24

essential fatty acid deficiency, 128

ethanol, 26*t*

ethylene oxide, 175

European Union: American apple ban (2012), 71; considering Roundup ban, 92

exercise: benefits of sweating during, 196, 204*t*; breathing, 179*t*, 189–90; health benefits of regular, 130; how beetroot juice impacts performance during, 186*fig*; how toxicity reduces ability to, 165; incorporate into your life regular, 218; slowing down Phase II detox with inadequate, 164; Type 2 diabetes associated with lack of, 36, 95

fabrics toxicity, 175, 216–17

fasting, 193. *See also* caloric restriction

fatigue: how toxins contribute to, 6; kidney disease and, 174; Sally's story on, 72–74; as symptom of increased lead levels, 53*t*; toxin interference with hormones causing, 25

Feldene, 132

fertilizer toxicity, 207

fiber: best supplements for, 99, 155; as critical to detoxification, 78–79, 101, 148, 179*t*; drinking water with, 120; fruit and vegetable sources of, 7, 83, 99; include more, 98; type 2 diabetes associated with lack of, 36

fish: mercury toxicity from, 26*t*, 86, 87*fig*; polychlorinated biphenyls (PCBs) toxicity from, 61; "wild-caught" versus farmed, 85–86

fish oil, 101, 142*t*, 165, 185

flame retardants toxicity, 175

flax oil, 101

Flint disaster (2014), 55–56

Flonase, 86

folic acid deficiency, 166

food additives, 175, 205*t*–6*t*

food allergies, 128, 131, 135

food coloring, 11, 80, 205*t*, 206*t*

food flavoring, 11, 80–81, 205*t*, 206*t*

food labels: learn to read and understand, 203–4; USDA Certified Organic, 204

foods: asparagusic acid–producing, 167–68; avoid additives and preservatives in, 203–4, 205*t*–6*t*; brassica-family, 98–99, 164, 165; choline-rich, 165; Clean 15 foods list of, 77, 97, 99–100, 189; cysteine-rich, 165; Dirty Dozen food list on, 71, 74, 88, 189, 203; easy tools for making health choices, 74; genetically modified organism (GMO), 6, 11, 53, 75, 91–92, 187; gluten-containing, 81–83; gluthathione producing, 141, 142*t*, 164; glycine-producing, 165; growing some of your own, 207; lactose intolerance to dairy, 83; loss of minerals in, 89*fig*–90; nutrient deficiency in, 89–93; organic, 71–74, 203; practicing toxin avoidance in, 10; primary sources of phosphates, 183*t*; promoting liver detoxification, 88, 98, 100, 120–22, 142*t*, 164; protein-rich, 85, 165, 182; rich in B vitamins, 164; Two-Week Jumpstart Diet, 98–101; Two-Week Kidney Detox Protocol, 179*t*, 185–88; Two-Week Liver Detox Protocol, 142*t*, 164. *See also* fruits; processed foods; vegetables

food toxins: contamination from, 6, 71–72; depression due to, 82–83; Dirty Dozen food list on, 71, 74, 88, 189, 203; genetically modified organism (GMO), 6, 11, 53, 75, 91–92; reducing your ingestion of, 43; reviewing the problem of, 70–72, 74–76; toxic overload due to different types of, 11; Two-Week Jumpstart Diet for eliminating, 45. *See also* pesticides toxicity; processed foods

formaldehyde, 213

"fracking" gas wells, 18

fruits: alkaline diet that includes lots of,

192; blueberries, 179*t*, 186, 187; Dirty Dozen food list on, 71, 74, 88; fiber from, 7, 83, 99; the healthiest, 88; Two-Week Jumpstart Diet, 100; Two-Week Kidney Detox Protocol, 179*t*; Two-Week Liver Detox Protocol, 142*t*, 164. *See also* foods

full-body detox (Week 9): caloric restriction during the, 192–93; green drinks, 192, 197–98; massage during, 192, 198–99; Roger's story on, 194–96; sending your body the right signals before, 191–92; taking saunas during the, 194, 195*t*, 196–97

furnishings toxicity, 216

GAIAM (www.experiencelife.com), 215
garlic, 120
gasoline (methyl tert-butyl ether, or MTBE), 175
gastrointestinal toxicity, 12*t*
gene expression damage, 24
genetically modified organism (GMO) foods: damage to the body by, 53; glyphosate herbicide used in, 187; increasing toxicity of, 6, 11, 75, 91–92
genetic variability: in adverse drug reactions (ADRs) and drug reactions, 168–69; in liver detoxification, 167–69; in toxin susceptibility of the liver, 29
giardia, 128
ginger, 185, 186
ginkgo biloba, 179*t*, 185, 186, 187
glutamine, 121
glutathione: activated intermediate toxin due to depleted stores of, 164; alcohol as depleting body's store of, 95, 132–33, 150; foods with cysteine for production of, 141, 142*t*, 164; how chemical toxins can deplete storage of, 110; how coffee impacts levels of, 101; how excess salt impairs ability to produce, 96; liver detoxification role of, 29, 95, 98, 142*t*, 158, 164, 166; supplement for, 29, 95, 142*t*; during Two-Week Liver Detox Protocol, 142*t*. *See also* supplements and vitamins
gluten-containing foods, 81–83
glycine-containing foods, 165

glyphosate herbicide, 187
goldenseal root power (*Hydrastis canadensis*), 114*t*, 119–20
gotu kola, 185, 186
grapefruit, 99
grapes, 74
Great Plains Laboratory, 96
green drinks, 192, 197–98
Grist website, 56
growth hormone, 195*t*
Gupta, Sanjay, 17–18
gut and digestive tract: alcohol impact on the, 131, 132–34*fig*; Conrad's story on, 109–12, 154; detoxification must always begin with, 108–9; endotoxins released by bacteria in, 112–13; healing the gut walls, 120–22; impact of bad bacteria on the, 115, 116–17; impact of toxic load on the, 107–8; interconnectivity with other organs of the body, 173; NSAIDs and damage to, 131*t*–32; probiotics for healthy, 98, 111–12, 113, 114*t*, 120; toxicity impact on, 114–15. *See also* the body; Two-Week Gut Protocol (Weeks 3 and 4)
gut bacteria: endotoxins released by, 112–13; impact on the gut by bad, 115, 116–17; probiotics to kill bad, 98, 111–12, 113, 114*t*, 120. *See also* leaky gut

HCBs toxins, 35*fig*, 86*fig*
HCHs toxins, 86*fig*
HDL cholesterol levels, 125
healing capacity, 3
healing crisis, 151
health: importance of detoxification to your, 36–37; liver detoxification affecting all aspects of, 140, 145; relationship between toxic exposures by age and impact on, 43*fig*; three key determinants for good, 9; Two-Week Jumpstart Diet and patients with poor, 105–6; understanding how toxins impact your, 1–2, 5–6, 39–41
health and beauty aids (HABAs): chemicals found in, 46*t*–49, 217; reducing your use of toxic, 10, 43, 204*t*, 217–18; toxic exposure and overload from, 6, 11, 45–49

health care: American Medical Association (AMA) influence over, 14, 145; failures of conventional, 21–22, 36; the practitioner's journey to new protocols of, 9–10. *See also* naturopathic medicine

heart disease. *See* cardiovascular heart disease

hematological toxicity: blood lead levels (BLLs), 51–52*fig*; blood-sugar problems due to, 5, 94*fig*, 105, 127*fig*–28; half-lives of typical toxins in the blood, 26*t*; symptoms of, 12*t*. *See also* blood

HEPA air filters, 204*t*, 213

herbicides toxicity, 15, 75, 91–92, 187, 207

herbs. *See* spices and herbs

HERMOSA study, 50

Herxheimer reaction, 151

hexachlorobutadiene, 175

hexachlorocyclopentadiene (HCCPD), 175

hiccups, 174

"hidden infections" fad, 129–30

high blood pressure (hypertension), 174, 180

high-fructose corn syrup (HFCS): impact on gut and digestive tract, 131, 134–35*fig*; NAFLD correlation to soda with, 129, 134–35*fig*; toxicity of, 93

home-building materials toxicity, 6

hormonal imbalances: HERMOSA study on reducing EDCs causing, 50; how toxins contribute to, 6; phthalates as endocrine disruptors causing, 31*t*, 47–48*fig*; thyroid, 25, 164, 208

hormones: how saunas increase production of growth, 195*t*; how toxins interfere with, 24–25; kidney detox of metabolites, 178

hot peppers, 74

house paint toxicity, 217

Huggins, Hal, 13

hypochlorhydria, 128

ibuprofen, 132

imidazolidinyl urea exposure, 46*t*

immune issues, 6

indole-3-carbinol, 142*t*

indomethacin, 132

industrial activities toxicity, 6

infants: prenatal mercury exposure in, 27; prenatal phthalates exposure to, 47–48*fig*; Teflon toxicity and low birth weight of, 208; toxic exposure through breast-feeding, 17, 61–62*fig*. *See also* children

infertility, 12*t*

inflammation: Charles's story on kidney detox and reducing, 182, 184–85; how toxins contribute to, 5; metabolic endotoxemia (ME) and, 129; overreactive, 117; quercetin for healing gut, 121; Teflon toxicity causing liver, 208

inflammatory bowel disease, 128

insomnia: kidney damage and, 174; symptom of increased lead levels, 53*t*

insulin resistance: endotoxin level related to, 125; metabolic endotoxemia (ME) and, 129

insulin sensitivity, 36

intense full-body detox (Week 9). *See* full-body detox (Week 9)

International Agency for Research on Cancer (IARC), 91

IQ decrease: as symptom of increased lead levels, 53*t*; as toxicity symptom, 19, 78, 88*fig*

irritable bowel syndrome, 128

itching (persistent), 174

Jack's story, 19–21

Jane's story, 117–18

Jennifer's story, 7–8

Johnson & Johnson lawsuit, 45

John's story, 129–30

Julie's story, 149–50

kale/collard greens, 74, 88

kidney dialysis, 138

kidney disease: chemical toxins that specifically target kidneys causing, 174–75; dialysis due to, 138; due to excessive protein in the diet, 182; Mayo Clinic on symptoms of, 174; toxic load that results in, 176; what causes loss of kidney function and, 176 kidney failure: as gradual process, 138–39; increasing phosphate levels associated with, 182; renal toxicity symptoms, 12*t*

kidneys: chemical toxins that specifically target the, 174–75; deterioration in function with aging, 180*fig*; filtration mechanism of the, 181*fig*; interconnectivity with other organs of the body, 173; leaky gut impact on, 109; what causes loss of function of the, 176. *See also* the body

kidneys detoxification: Charles's story on, 182, 184–85; Conrad's story on, 109–11, 154; filtering blood by the kidneys for, 175–76, 179–81*fig*; how alcohol weakens capacity for, 95–96; three ways kidneys excrete toxics, 181; water drinking recommendation during, 98, 179*fig*, 189. *See also* detoxification; Two-Week Kidney Detox Protocol (Weeks 7 and 8)

kiwi fruit, 99

Kristof, Nicholas, 18

lactase enzyme, 83

Lactobacillus species, 114*t*, 120

lactose intolerance, 83, 84

law-enforcement meth exposure, 175–76

lead exposure: ALS risk associated with, 31*t*; bone loss due to, 7, 24; Connie's story on, 54–55; detoxification through saunas, 195*t*; Flint disaster (2014) of, 55–56; HABAs and, 48–49; half-life in blood, 26*t*; impact on IQ points, 19; lead-removal support protocol to reduce, 7–8; Roman Empire decline due to, 23; symptoms in children and adults, 52–53*t*

leaky gut: association between other diseases and, 124–28; bad bacteria and toxins causing, 116–17; excessive consumption of alcohol cause of, 131, 132–34*fig*; food allergies and, 128, 131, 135; health consequences of, 122–24, 127*fig*–28; HFCS impact on, 131, 134–35*fig*; high-fructose corn syrup (HFCS) and, 131, 134–35*fig*; how toxins contribute

to, 5; NSAIDs causing, 131*t*–32; wide prevalence of, 114. *See also* gut bacteria; organ damage

licorice (DGL, deglycyrrhizinated licorice), 121–22

liver: acetaminophen toxicity causing failure of the, 170; BPA levels clogging the, 5; genetic variability in toxin susceptibility and detox of, 29, 167–69; HPCS impact on the, 93; interconnectivity with other organs of the body, 173; leaky gut impact on the, 109, 113, 123–24, 125–26*fig*; nonalcoholic fatty liver disease (NAFLD) of, 129; producing enzymes that break down toxic chemicals, 100, 101, 147, 148–49, 155–60; soda consumption and NAFLD, 134–35*fig*; Teflon toxicity and inflammation of the, 208. *See also* the body

liver detoxification: of acetaminophen (Tylenol), 169–70, 171*fig*; adjusting the rate of, 154–55; age differences and capacity for, 166; all aspects of health and disease risk impacted by, 140, 145; dandelion, artichoke, and turmeric herbs to help, 152; extra supports for weak capacity for, 170–72; fiber as critical to, 78–79, 101, 148; foods that promote, 88, 98, 100, 120–22, 142*fig*, 164; genetic variability in, 167–69; glutathione antioxidant helping with, 29, 95, 98, 142*t*, 158, 164; how alcohol weakens capacity for, 95–96; inhibitors during, 163*t*; Julie's story on, 149–50; liver enzymes to break down toxic chemicals for, 100, 101, 147, 148–49, 155–60; liver's filtering the blood for, 147, 148; liver's production of bile for, 147, 148; natural process of, 123; pathways during the, 156*fig*; self-assessing your experience with, 151–53; Susan's story on, 146–47; symptoms to watch out for during, 155; symptom survey on, 152; understanding the process of, 143–45, 153–54. *See also* detoxification; Two-Week Liver Detox Protocol (Weeks 5 and 6)

liver enzymes: activated intermediate modified toxin produced by incomplete detox by, 164; metabolic process of Phase I detoxification by, 157–60, 164; produced by body to break down toxic chemicals, 100, 101, 147, 148–49; the science behind detoxification by, 155–56; sulfoxidase, 168
low birth weight, 208
low energy. *See* fatigue
low-protein diet, 166
lung cancer risk, 31*t*
Lustig, Robert H., 72

magnesium citrate, 179*t*
Malkan, Stacy, 49
mangoes, 99
Maria's story, 83–84
marijuana, 95, 209
massage, 192, 198–99
Maybelline, 48
Mayo Clinic, 174
meal plans: Toxin Solution Maintenance Plan, 210*t*–12*t*; Two-Week Jumpstart Diet, 101, 102*t*–4*t*; Two-Week Liver Detox Protocol, 143*t*
medical care. *See* health care; naturopathic medicine
medications: acetaminophen (Tylenol), 86, 169–70; adverse drug reactions (ADRs) to, 168–69; antibiotics, 86; genetic variability in reactions to, 168–69; natural therapies versus, 132; nonsteroidal anti-inflammatory drugs (NSAIDs), 131*t*–32; NSAIDs (nonsteroidal anti-inflammatory drugs), 131*t*–32
memory loss, 53*t*
menstrual cycle disruption, 12*t*
mental sharpness. *See* cognition
mercury exposure: amalgams ("silver fillings") source of, 25–26*t*, 27; bone loss due to, 7; burning contaminated coal source of, 18; detoxification protocol for, 7–8; detoxification through saunas, 195*t*; fish and, 26*t*, 86, 87*t*; half-life in blood, 26*t*; impact on IQ points, 19; "mad hatter disease" due to, 23; Minamata (Japan)

water contamination, 190; prenatal, 27; sources of and risks for, 25–27
metabolic endotoxemia (ME), 128, 129–30, 134
metabolic processes: description of the, 157; of liver enzymes breaking down toxins, 157–60
metabolic syndrome: synergistic effects of toxins on, 29–30*fig*; toxic exposures, age, and, 43*t*; toxin levels correlation with, 35*fig*. *See also* obesity
metabolism disruption, 127*fig*
metabolites: description and functions of, 115; detoxification through saunas, 195*t*; endotoxin, 112–13, 123–24, 133; kidney detox of hormone, 178; phthalates, 31*t*, 47–48*fig*, 52–53, 195*t*, 213, 217; understanding, 115–16
methamphetamine exposure, 195*t*
Michigan State University, 22
microcirculation: beetroot juice benefits for, 186*fig*; foods, herbs, and spices benefiting kidney, 185–88; herbal medicines to improve, 185; kidney damage related to, 180. *See also* blood
migraine, 128
Mildred's story, 43–45
Minamata (Japan) methyl mercury contamination, 190
mineral loss in foods (1941–1991), 89*fig*
miscarriages, 12*t*
mitochondrial disorders, 6, 124, 164, 175
mold toxicity: black mold, 6, 214; VOCs (volatile organic compounds) in house paints and, 217
molybdenum deficiency, 167
monosodium glutamate (MSG), 80–81
Monsanto Corporation lawsuit, 58
Morello, Gaetano, 207
multivitamins, 142*t*, 179*t*, 186

NAC (n-acetyl cysteine), 142*t*, 150, 165, 179*t*
NAFLD (nonalcoholic fatty liver disease), 129, 134–35*fig*
NAPQI (N-acetyl-p-benzoquinone imine), 170

naproxen, 132

natural cleansers, 215–16

Natural Factors, 99, 198

Natural Resources Defense Council (NRDC), 213

naturopathic medicine: conventional medicine's attempts to suppress, 14, 145; decreasing your toxic load using, 10, 11; description and focus of, 11; medical philosophy and secret strength of, 64; toxicity and detoxification protocols of, 15. *See also* health care

nausea: as kidney damage symptom, 174; as sign of toxicity, 6, 12*t*; as symptom of too rapid detox, 155

nectarines, 74

neurological toxicity symptoms, 12*t*

n-hexane exposure, 6

Nine-Week Toxin Solution: intense full-body detox (Week 9), 191–99; introduction to the nine week, 10, 49–50; neutralizing and releasing toxins during, 40; preparing physically and psychologically for, 138; recommended for everyone, 40; releasing toxins during the, 49–50; Toxin Solution Maintenance Plan after the, 202–19; Two-Week Gut Protocol (Weeks 3 and 4), 109–14*t*, 117–39; Two-Week Jumpstart Diet (Weeks 1 and 2), 69–74, 78–79, 97–106; Two-Week Kidney Detox Protocol (Weeks 7 and 8), 171–90; Two-Week Liver Detox Protocol (Weeks 5 and 6), 140–72; why you might not notice improvement midway through the, 137–39

nitric oxide, 186

nitrosodiphenylamine, 175

nonalcoholic fatty liver disease (NAFDL), 129, 134–35*fig*

Noreen's story, 93–94*fig*

NSAIDs (nonsteroidal anti-inflammatory drugs), 131*t*–32

nutritional deficiencies: how Phase II liver detoxification is stalled by, 166; mineral loss in foods (1941–1991), 89*fig*; Two-Week Jumpstart Diet designed to correct, 166; vitamin D deficiency, 133

obesity: diabetes risk of toxins versus, 36; gut toxins and, 124–25; increasing rates of, 12, 78; John's story on, 129–30; kidney detox capacity lowered by, 180; metabolic endotoxemia (ME) and, 129; Noreen's story on, 93–94*fig*; toxicity and childhood, 18. *See also* metabolic syndrome

OCPs (organochlorine pesticides), 4

oils recommendations, 101

onion (*Alluim* genus), 99, 120

OPs (organophosphates), 53, 78, 88*fig*

Oregon State University, 22

organ damage: how toxins cause, 24; to the kidneys, 138, 138–39, 174–76, 182; to the liver, 5, 93, 129, 134–35*fig*, 170, 208. *See also* leaky gut

organic foods: apples, 71–72; CSA (community-supported agriculture) to purchase, 203; reducing toxic exposure through, 72; Sally's story on switching to, 72–74; Toxin Solution Maintenance Plan on continuing to eat, 203; USDA Certified Organic labels of, 204

OSHA (Occupational Safety and Health Administration), 19–20

osteoporosis, 7, 24, 90

oxychlordane, 35*fig*

OxyContin, 86

P5P (pyridoxal-5-phosphate) supplement, 132

PAHs (polycyclic aromatic hydrocarbons), 31*t*

papayas, 99

parabens exposure, 46*t*

Parkinson's disease, 71, 143

patient stories: Charles's, 182, 184–85; Connie's, 54–55; Conrad's, 109–12, 154; Ed's, 82–83; Jack's, 19–21; Jane's, 117–18; Jennifer's, 7–8; John's, 129–30; Julie's, 149–50; Maria's, 83–84; Mildred's, 43–45; Noreen's, 93–94*fig*; Peter's and Don's, 15–16; Roger's, 194–96; Sally's, 72–74; Susan's, 146–47

Paxil, 86

PBDEs (polybrominated diphenyl ethers): fish contamination of, 84*fig*; our everyday exposure to, 4; select clothing without, 217

PCBs (polychlorinated biphenyls): age and accumulation of, 61*fig*, 62–65; detoxification through saunas, 195*t*; fish contaminated with, 85, 86*fig*; half-life in blood, 26*t*; how they build over a lifetime, 62–65; impact of exposure to, 60–62; origins and banning of, 58, 60*fig*; our everyday exposure to, 4, 58, 59–60; risk of diseases associated with, 31*t*, 35*fig*

peaches, 74

perfluoroalkyls, 175

perfluorochemicals, 216

Pesticide Information Project of Cooperative Extension Offices, 22

pesticides toxicity: ADHD risk and, 31*t*, 88; DDT, 26*t*, 31*t*, 35*fig*, 85, 86*fig*; everyday exposure to, 15, 17, 19; impact on food by, 72; OCPs (organochlorine pesticides), 4; OPs (organophosphates), 53, 78, 88*fig*; risk for dementia associated with, 88*fig*; risk of disease due to specific toxins, 31*t*; Sally's story on, 72–74; Sheryl's story on, 76–78; specifically targeting the kidneys, 175; synergistic effects of, 29–30*fig*; worsen metabolic syndrome and diabetes, 29–30, 35*fig*. *See also* chemical toxicity; food toxins

Peter's story, 15

petroleum hydrocarbons, 175

PFASs (perfluorinated alkylated substances), 16–17, 195*t*

PFCs (perfluorinated chemicals), 4

PGX supplement, 99, 155

phenlyenediamine (Cl+number), 46*t*

phosphates: all-cause mortality association with excessive intake of, 184*fig*; kidney failure and excessive consumption of, 182; phosphate ester flame retardants, 175; primary food sources of, 183*t*

phthalates: associated with diabetes risk, 31*t*; caution against air fresheners that release, 213; damage to the body by, 52–53;

detoxification through saunas, 195*t*; HABAs and toxicity of, 47–48*fig*, 217

pineapples, 99

Pizzorno, Joseph: four-generation photograph with, 66*fig*; his journey to practice of detoxification, 13–15; lessons learned from four generations, 65–68; motorcycle-touring, Australia (2015), 67*fig*; *Total Wellness* written by, 202

plastic packaged food, 207–8

pollutants: benzene, 3–4, 26*t*, 213; formaldehyde, 213; "fracking" gas wells source of, 18; OCPs (organochlorine pesticides), 4; OPs (organophosphates), 53, 78, 88*fig*; PAHs (polycyclic aromatic hydrocarbons), 31*t*; PBDEs (polybrominated diphenyl ethers), 4, 84*fig*; PCBs (polychlorinated biphenyls), 4, 26*t*, 31*t*, 35*fig*, 58, 59–65, 85, 86*fig*, 195*t*; PFASs (perfluorinated alkylated substances), 16–17, 195*t*; PFCs (perfluorinated chemicals), 4; POPs (persistent organic pollutants), 85, 101, 175, 178, 195*t*; VOCs (volatile organic compounds), 4, 213, 216, 217

POPs (persistent organic pollutants): detoxification through saunas, 195*t*; fish contaminated with, 85; fish oils with, 101; kidney detox of, 178; specifically targeting the kidneys, 175

Portland arsenic and cadmium exposure, 56–58

potatoes, 74

President's National Cancer Panel (2010), 13, 17

probiotics: to kill bad gut bacteria, 98, 111–12; repairing the gut with, 113, 114*t*, 120, 136

processed foods: do not buy food packaged in plastic, 207–8; as don'ts, 79; food preservatives and additives in, 175, 205*t*–6*t*; nutrient deficiency in, 89–93; read food labels of, 203–4; sources of phosphates in, 183*t*; toxicity of, 80–81. *See also* foods; food toxins

Procter & Gamble, 48

propylene glycol, 175

protein: alkaline diet limiting your animal, 189–90, 192; diet of low, 166; foods rich in, 85, 165, 182; kidney damage due to diet of excessive, 182

psoriasis, 128

Pure Synergy Superfood, 198

pyridoxal-5-phosphate (PSP) supplements, 132

quaternium-15 exposure, 46t

quercetin, 121

rashes: alcoholism and, 133; kidney damage and, 12t

recreational drugs, 95

renal toxicity symptoms, 12t

reproductive toxicity symptoms, 12t

research. See toxicity research

respiratory toxicity symptoms, 12t

Revlon, 48

Rey, Bill, 13

rheumatoid arthritis: Jane's story on, 117–18; leaky gut and, 113, 128; Mildred's story on, 43–45

Rhode Island Hospital, 71

Roger's story, 194–96

Roman Empire decline, 23

Roundup (herbicide), 92, 207

saccharin, 81

safe cleaning products, 215–16

Sally's story, 72–74

salt: decreasing your consumption of, 179t; kidney detox of, 178; toxicity of, 96, 206t

saunas: the best way to take, 196–97; detoxification through, 195t; different cultures that practice, 194; during intense full-body detox week, 195, 196

seizures, 53t

selenium supplement, 166

Shakespeare, William, 14

shortness of breath, 174

Silent Spring (Carson), 17

"singer's voice" treatment, 122

sleep problems: kidney damage and, 174;

symptom of increased lead levels, 53t

smoke alarms, 204t, 214

smoking cigarettes, 31t

snap peas, 74

sodas: artificial sweeteners in, 11, 81, 93, 205t, 206t; correlation between fatty liver disease and, 135fig; HFCS used in, 93, 129, 134–35fig; NAFLD and, 129, 134–35fig

solvent toxicity: detoxification through saunas, 195t; Jack's story on, 19–21; Julie's story on, 149–50; kidney damage through, 175; using natural cleansers that do not have, 215–16; Roger's story on, 194–96

soy products toxicity, 90–92

spices and herbs: ginger, 185, 186; ginkgo biloba, 179t, 185, 186, 187; goldenseal root power (Hydrastis canadensis), 114t, 119–20; gotu kola, 185; turmeric, 100, 142t, 152, 185, 186, 187; Two-Week Jumpstart Diet, 100; Two-Week Kidney Detox Protocol, 179t; Two-Week Liver Detox Protocol, 142t, 164

spinach: cadmium toxicity in, 90; Dirty Dozen food, 74, 88

Splenda, 81

stories. See patient stories

strawberries, 74

stroke: conversion of dietary choline to toxic TMA causing, 125, 126fig; gut endotoxins and, 127fig; metabolic endotoxemia (ME) and, 129

sugar: conversion of dietary polysaccharides to, 124; diabetes epidemic caused by toxins versus, 32fig–35fig; health issues associated with, 92–93; increasing consumption (1822–2005), 33fig. See also artificial sweeteners

sulfoxidase (liver enzyme), 168

supplements and vitamins: anthocyanins, 185; artichoke extract, 142t, 152; curcumin, 142t, 179t, 186, 187; dandelion, 142t, 152; DGL (deglycyrrhizinated licorice), 121–22; for fiber, 99, 155; fish oil, 101, 142t,

supplements and vitamins *(continued)*
165, 185; ginkgo biloba, 179*t*; indole-3-
carbinol, 142*t*; liver detoxification herbal
defenders, 142*t*, 152; magnesium citrate,
179*t*; molybdenum, 167; multivitamin,
142*t*, 179*t*, 186; NAC (n-acetyl cysteine),
142*t*, 150, 165, 179*t*; P5P (pyridoxal-5-
phosphate), 132; PGX, 99, 155; pyridoxal-
5-phosphate (PSP), 132; selenium, 166;
turmeric, 100, 142*t*, 152, 185; Two-Week
Gut Protocol, 121–22; Two-Week Kidney
Detox Protocol, 179*t*; Two-Week Liver
Detox Protocol, 142*t*, 166–67; vitamin B,
142*t*, 164, 165, 166–67, 178; vitamin C,
142*t*, 165, 167; vitamin D, 133. *See also*
glutathione
Susan's story, 146–47
sweet bell peppers, 74
sweet corn, 99
sweet peas, 99
sweet potatoes, 99
swelling of feet/ankles, 174
Symptom survey, 152
Synergy Company, 198

Tagamet, 86
Tartrazine dye, 80
Teflon cookware, 208
Teflon flu, 208
Think Dirty app, 46
thyroid hormone imbalance, 25, 164, 208
toluene, 26*t*
tomatoes, 74
Total Wellness (Pizzorno), 202
toxic damage: body dysregulation, 22–23;
the body's 155-160 stores protection
from, 29, 158; eight ways that our bodies
experience, 23–25; by gut toxins, 124–28;
how disease is related to, 1–2, 5–6,
23–25; repairing the, 10; symptoms in
children and adults of lead-related, 52–53*t*
toxic exposure: account for synergistic
effects of, 29–32; conducting more
long-term research on, 28; examples of
mass, 55–58; examples of minimizing
your, 3–4; extent of your, 9; failure of

conventional medicine to address, 21–22;
lessons learned form four generations on,
65–68; mercury and lead, 7–8; as part of
our everyday life, 3–7, 16–19; relationship
between age, health challenges, and,
43*fig*; Toxic Troubleshooter to assess your,
41–43; tracking all, 27–28; why it is hard
to avoid sources of, 6, 16–17, 50–53*t*,
64–65
toxicity research: HERMOSA study,
50; need for more long-term, 28; on
synergistic interaction of toxins, 30*fig*–31;
on VOCs in house paints and mold
toxicity, 217
toxic load: ability of your body to neutralize
or excrete toxins, 9; breast-feeding
decreases woman's, 61–62*fig*; easy ways
to reduce your, 43; gut bacteria's released
endotoxins adding to, 112–13; impact
on gut and digestive tract, 107–8; on the
kidneys, 176; naturopathic medicine to
reduce, 10, 11; the practitioner's journey
to new protocols for reducing, 9–10;
synergistic effects of, 29–32. *See also*
detoxification
toxic overload: characteristics of, 11–12;
symptoms and general types of toxicity
and, 12*t*
Toxic Troubleshooter: assessing toxic
exposures using the, 41–42; how to
effectively use the, 42–43, 171
toxins: activated intermediate, 164;
consumer-product, 12; disease risk due
to specific, 31*t*–32; distinguishing
between avoidable and unavoidable,
39–40; endotoxins, 112–13, 123–24;
identify individual variations in susceptibility to, 29; interacting with other health
environment factors, 2; understanding how
they impact your health, 1–2, 5–6, 39–41
Toxin Solution Maintenance Plan:
continue getting out the old toxins,
218–19; eat organically grown food, 203;
recommendations for the, 204*t*; strategies
for keeping new toxins from your body,
202–18; three goals of the, 202

Toxin Solution. *See* Nine-Week Toxin
    Solution
Transatlantic Trade and Investment
    Partnership (TTIP), 71
triclosan exposure, 46*t*
trimethylamine (TMA) toxin, 125, 126*fig*
trimethylamine-N-oxide (TMAO)
    toxin, 125
turmeric, 100, 142*t*, 152, 185, 186, 187
Two-Week Gut Protocol (Weeks 3 and 4):
    Conrad's story on, 109–12, 154; Jane's
    story on, 117–18; John's story on, 129–30;
    step 1: kill the bad bacteria of the gut, 113,
    114*t*, 119–20; step 2: repair the gut, 114*t*,
    120; step 3: introduce health bacteria
    and repair gut walls, 113, 114*t*, 120, 136;
    step 4: stop the damage from recurring,
    131*t*–35*fig*, 136. *See also* gut and digestive
    tract
Two-Week Jumpstart Diet (Weeks 1 and
    2): designed to correct most nutritional
    deficiencies, 166; the don'ts of, 79–82;
    the do's during your, 97–101; easy tools
    for making health food choices, 74;
    getting ready to begin the, 69–70, 78–79;
    maintenance diet versus detoxification of,
    106; the maybes during, 101; meal plans
    for the, 101, 102*t*–4*t*; what to expect
    during, 104–5; who requires medical
    supervision for, 105–6
Two-Week Kidney Detox Protocol (Weeks
    7 and 8): alkalinizing your tissues during,
    189–90; Charles's story on, 182, 184–85;
    foods and supplements during the, 179*t*,
    185–88; improving microcirculation
    during, 185–87; review of kidney cleanse
    during, 190; the two things that will
    happen during the, 176–77; understand-
    ing the process of, 177–79; water drinking
    recommendation during, 98, 179*fig*, 189.
    See also kidneys detoxification
Two-Week Liver Detox Protocol (Phase I):
    detoxification pathways during, 156*fig*;
    foods to eat to promote a successful, 88,
    98, 100, 120–22, 142*t*, 164; liver enzymes
    and interaction between Phase II and,

155–56, 164; metabolic process of liver
    enzymes breaking down toxins during,
    157–60
Two-Week Liver Detox Protocol (Phase II):
    amino acids required for liver enzymes
    work during, 140; conjugation process
    during the, 126; detoxification pathways
    during, 156*fig*; extra supports for weak
    detox capacity during, 170–72; getting
    rid of NAPQI during, 170; key nutrients
    required for successful, 165; liver enzymes
    and interaction between Phase I and,
    155–56, 164; what can stall the, 166–67
Two-Week Liver Detox Protocol (Weeks 5
    and 6): description of the, 3, 10, 141–42*t*;
    foods and supplements during, 142*t*; goals
    of the, 141; Phase I and Phase II of the, 88,
    98, 100, 120–22, 141–72; sample menu
    plans, 143*t*. *See also* liver detoxification
Tylenol (acetaminophen): detoxification of,
    169–70, 171*fig*; toxicity of, 86, 170
Type 1 diabetes: endotoxins connected to,
    123; HABAs toxicity associated with risk
    of, 218; increasing rates of, 12; leaky gut
    association with, 113; polychlorinated
    biphenyls (PCBs) exposure and, 63;
    specific toxins associated with risk of,
    31*t*, 35*fig*, 40; sugar versus toxins as cause
    of epidemic of, 32*fig*–35*fig*; synergistic
    effects of toxins on, 29–30*fig*; toxic
    exposures, age, and, 43*t*; Two-Week
    Jumpstart Diet medical supervision for
    people with, 105–6. *See also* blood-sugar
    levels; diseases
Type 2 diabetes: causes of prediabetes
    and, 95, 128; combination of causes
    and mechanisms of, 36, 71, 78, 128;
    endotoxins connected to, 123; HABAs
    toxicity associated with risk of, 218; leaky
    gut association with, 113; metabolic
    endotoxemia (ME) and, 129; Noreen's
    story on, 93–94*fig*; population diagnosed
    with (1958–2009), 32*fig*; Two-Week
    Jumpstart Diet medical supervision for
    people with, 105–6. *See also* blood-sugar
    levels; diseases

University of California Davis, 22
University of California San Francisco, 72
University of Pittsburgh, 18
University of Washington School of
    Medicine, 14
urine: alkalinizing your, 189; kidney damage
    and changes in, 12t, 174; kidney detox
    and color of, 178
USDA Certified Organic label, 204

vaccination mercury contamination, 26t
Valium, 86
vegetables: alkaline diet that includes lots of,
    192; Clean 15 foods list, 77, 97, 99–100;
    creasing brassica-family and healthy,
    98–99; Dirty Dozen food list on, 71, 74,
    88; fiber from, 7, 83, 99; green drinks
    made from, 192, 197–98; the healthiest,
    88; Two-Week Jumpstart Diet, 99–100;
    Two-Week Kidney Detox Protocol, 179t;
    Two-Week Liver Detox Protocol, 142t,
    164. See also fruits
Vioxx, 132
vitamin B, 142t, 164, 165, 166–67, 178
vitamin C, 142t, 165, 167
vitamin D deficiency, 133
VOCs (volatile organic compounds), 4, 213,
    216, 217
vomiting: as kidney damage symptom, 174;
    as sign of toxicity, 12t

water contamination: arsenic, 18, 96;
    Connie's story on, 54–55; Flint
    disaster (2014), 55–56; mercury, 26t;
    Minamata (Japan) methyl mercury,
    190; OCPs (organochlorine pesticides),
    4; PBDEs (polybrominated diphenyl
    ethers), 4, 84fig; PCBs (polychlorinated
    biphenyls), 4, 26t, 31t, 35fig, 58, 59–65,
    85, 86fig, 195t; PFASs (perfluorinated
    alkylated substances), 16–17, 195t; PFCs
    (perfluorinated chemicals), 4; POPs
    (persistent organic pollutants), 85, 101,
    175, 178, 195t; strategies for avoiding,
    96–97
water drinking: chlorination of our,
    214; clean water for, 189; four quarts
    recommendation, 98, 179fig, 189
water supplies: chlorination of our, 214;
    filter your cooking and bathing, 204t;
    resources for testing your, 96, 214;
    strategies to ensure safe, 96–97,
    213–14
World Health Organization, 81
World's Healthiest Foods (www.WHFoods
    .org), 209

xylenes, 6, 175

zinc deficiency, 166
Zoloft, 86